Preparing to sit
the FRCA

BMA

D1628300

WITHDRAWN
FROM LIBRARY
BRITISH MEDICAL ASSOCIATION

1000458

Preparing to Pass the FRCA
Strategies for exam success

Dr Caroline Whymark MB ChB FRCA
Consultant Anaesthetist
University Hospital Crosshouse
Kilmarnock
Scotland, UK

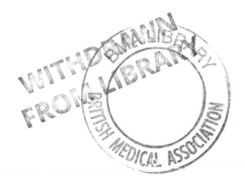

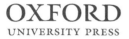
OXFORD
UNIVERSITY PRESS

Great Clarendon Street, Oxford, OX2 6DP,
United Kingdom

Oxford University Press is a department of the University of Oxford.
It furthers the University's objective of excellence in research, scholarship,
and education by publishing worldwide. Oxford is a registered trade mark of
Oxford University Press in the UK and in certain other countries

© Oxford University Press 2016

The moral rights of the author have been asserted

First Edition published in 2016

Impression: 1

All rights reserved. No part of this publication may be reproduced, stored in
a retrieval system, or transmitted, in any form or by any means, without the
prior permission in writing of Oxford University Press, or as expressly permitted
by law, by licence or under terms agreed with the appropriate reprographics
rights organization. Enquiries concerning reproduction outside the scope of the
above should be sent to the Rights Department, Oxford University Press, at the
address above

You must not circulate this work in any other form
and you must impose this same condition on any acquirer

Published in the United States of America by Oxford University Press
198 Madison Avenue, New York, NY 10016, United States of America

British Library Cataloguing in Publication Data

Data available

Library of Congress Control Number: 2015955004

ISBN 978-0-19-874868-7

Printed and bound by
Ashford Colour Press Ltd.

Oxford University Press makes no representation, express or implied, that the
drug dosages in this book are correct. Readers must therefore always check
the product information and clinical procedures with the most up-to-date
published product information and data sheets provided by the manufacturers
and the most recent codes of conduct and safety regulations. The authors and
the publishers do not accept responsibility or legal liability for any errors in the
text or for the misuse or misapplication of material in this work. Except where
otherwise stated, drug dosages and recommendations are for the non-pregnant
adult who is not breast-feeding

Links to third party websites are provided by Oxford in good faith and
for information only. Oxford disclaims any responsibility for the materials
contained in any third party website referenced in this work.

Preface

I first became aware that the pass rate in FRCA exams was below the national average in my region, the West of Scotland, in 2009. I began to think of why this may be and how it could be improved. From my experience in teaching and training, I knew that exam candidates were highly intelligent professionals, often very good at their job, with a past history of exam and academic success—yet many could not pass the FRCA.

Success in the FRCA exams is not only related to knowledge of anaesthesia and the exam syllabus. In addition, a variety of skills are required, including many life skills such as prioritization, delegation, self-motivation, and stress management. The attitude of individuals and their departments towards exams has a significant bearing on the outcome of exam sittings, to the extent that some would say that the FRCA is predominately a test of one's life management skills rather than the sum total of one's knowledge.

Management of the entire process of taking exams is not widely taught, yet the ability to do this alongside a demanding professional role and important commitments outwith the hospital is integral to exam success. I developed a regional course to address this issue and began delivering it in January 2011. The focus is not on teaching knowledge per se but centres, instead, upon preparing the candidate to present those parts of their knowledge specifically asked for, in the format required by each element of the exam, and to facilitate real-time, repeated practice of doing so.

The regional course forms the basis of this book, and both emphasize all that must be done to ensure that an intelligent doctor who has studied the syllabus can ultimately pass the FRCA.

Caroline Whymark, 2015

Disclaimer

The advice and opinions expressed in this book are my own and are based on the experience I have gained in this field over a decade of helping anaesthetists in training prepare for exams. Of note, I am not an examiner for the Royal College of Anaesthetists and have no input into the development of any element of the FRCA. Indeed if this was the case, a conflict of roles would have precluded development of both the course and a book of this nature.

The content of this book does not reflect the views of the Royal College of Anaesthetists nor has it been endorsed by them. However, much of the information contained within this guide is available on their website (http://www.rcoa.ac.uk), including the curriculum to which the exams and this book relate.

C.W.

Contents

Detailed Contents

PART 1

THE ESSENTIALS

CHAPTER 1

Introduction to adult learning and postgraduate exams

I am always ready to learn although I do not always like being taught

Winston Churchill

CONTENTS

Postgraduate exams are a significant hurdle to overcome in order to progress through postgraduate training and gain a Certificate of Completion of Training (CCT). They are the gateway to becoming a consultant. However, studying for postgraduate exams is an onerous task. To pass requires a great breadth and depth of knowledge and the ability to present it in the correct format for each component of the exams. There are many courses and resources which impart the knowledge required, but the supporting facets required for effective exam preparation and presentation are often neglected. Knowledge alone is not enough to ensure success in the Fellowship of the Royal College of Anaesthetists (FRCA) and we each know excellent anaesthetists of all grades who found it difficult to pass exams. This book will help you study effectively and maximize your performance in exams.

The opportunity cost

There is a significant failure rate for all postgraduate exams, making them costly in terms of money as well as time (that is, both time to spend on leisure and social pursuits is curtailed and time spent in training may be prolonged).

Further, learning and studying as an adult is difficult: it takes longer, and is very different to being at school or university. The FRCA exams present themselves at a time in life when studying is no longer the sole priority for candidates. Most have established commitments and other demands on their time. Exam preparation must occur alongside clinical shift working, and fit in with children and responsibilities for child care or care of increasingly dependent elderly relatives. In addition, consideration must be given to partners and their careers too. Some doctors may be significantly involved in pursuits outside of medicine and anaesthesia, such as sport or music. Having other aspects of life to consider makes it much harder to focus on revision and preparation to the exclusion of everything else. Difficult and perhaps unpopular decisions with friends and family have to be made, and time spent in other areas may have to be sacrificed in order to prioritize

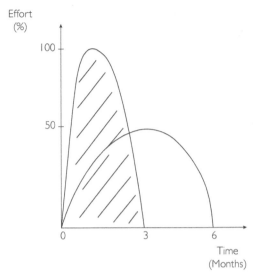

Figure 1.1 It is difficult to maintain maximal effort for an extended period of time.

study and exam success. The associated guilt resulting from these choices becomes something else to deal with.

Do not forget, however, that all these changes and hardships need exist only for a few months for those who are serious about passing the exams. By doing everything possible to make the first attempt at each component of the exam the best it can possibly be, you will maximize your chance of success and minimize the duration of time that studying and exams take over your life, as shown in the effort–time graph in Figure 1.1. Here, the area under each curve is constant and represents the work to be done to pass the exam. Curve A (shaded) over three months shows a far preferable way of working than curve B over six months.

Do not ever 'have a go' at a postgraduate exam to 'see if you can get it'. You will not. Instead, you will begin a psychological cycle of failure, making subsequent attempts more difficult. Of course, there will be those exceptions to this rule, and you may know some of them. It pays to remember though that most people *are* the rule, rather than the exception to it.

Unfortunately, as we get older, learning occurs more slowly and so takes longer. The stakes are different too. Prior exams have assessed whether we were suitable for a career in medicine, then for training in anaesthesia, both occurring at a time where many other options remained open to us. By the time candidates sit the final FRCA, most will have invested several years training in anaesthesia and are required to pass this exam to complete that training. Failure at this stage leaves individuals with severely limited options, especially now that changing specialty is very difficult. Thus, the stakes are high and the pressure to pass is significant.

Managing stress

Stress is an inevitable part of postgraduate exams. It is said to occur when one's normal coping methods are inadequate to deal with the problems presented. You cannot control the number of stressors affecting you but you can control your reaction to them. Being able to do so is one of the covert ways in which the exams assess your ability to perform in stressful, senior, high-stakes situations. A degree of stress can improve productivity and performance, but a continual increase will eventually overwhelm an individual's ability to cope and it then becomes paralysing

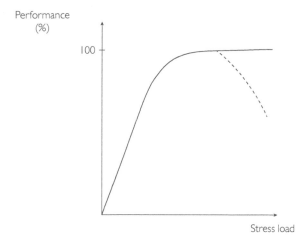

Figure 1.2 Stress improves performance up to a point before additional stress becomes detrimental.

and detrimental to performance on many counts. This occurs in a manner not dissimilar to Starling's Law of the heart which relates stroke volume with increasing end diastolic volume, as shown in Figure 1.2. As our stress load increases, so does performance, until our coping systems are saturated and begin to decompensate or fail, at which point performance begins to suffer.

Getting help

There are many sources of help available to exam candidates which you should be prepared to ask for. Consultants in your department will do everything they can to help you succeed. Do not forget that they have all been in the same position. Other trainees can become study buddies. You can ask for support at home. Attend courses targeting the exam, if possible, but ensure these are re-vision for you—do not rely on them to cover all the material you have not yet got around to studying. There is little benefit in transferring the content of lecturers' slides to your notebook if it completely bypasses your brain! This type of knowledge learning can be achieved through self study and reading books or other materials. Ideally, however, it will occur through clinical exposure, allowing you to see what you are learning in action and being able to question your consultant trainer at the time. This makes your learning much more memorable and easier to recall.

Making it happen

The bottom line is that it all comes down to you. *You* must do the work and *you* must sit and pass the exam. No-one can do this for you. You have the ability to pass the FRCA but whether or not you do depends on how much you want to pass and how much effort you are prepared to put into ensuring that you do. It is not easy to pass postgraduate exams but it is possible. Many can and do succeed, despite having a concurrent tumultuous period in their life. It is important to take a long-term view. The rewards are a passage into higher and advanced training, a CCT, and a consultant career with security and opportunity not seen in business, banking, or even other grades of hospital doctoring. Six months of hard work to the exclusion of everything else seems a small price to pay.

This book will show you how to incorporate studying into your life and motivate yourself to prepare for and pass the FRCA.

CHAPTER 2

Motivation

Discipline is the bridge between goals and accomplishment . . . we must all suffer . . . the pain of discipline or the pain of regret and disappointment

Jim Rohn (self-help guru and personal development pioneer)

CONTENTS

Adult learners have to be self-motivated to study and learn. No-one checks whether revision is being done or not, no-one insists you do it, and no-one forces you to sit these exams. Every candidate wants to pass and yet, despite this, many find it hard to motivate themselves sufficiently to achieve the level of studying required. Lack of motivation and lack of self belief are psychological barriers to success and you must learn to control your mind and manage negative thoughts and attitudes. Negative responses must be 'unlearned' and replaced with positive management strategies and a positive mental attitude. If you continually state and believe that you 'are rubbish and always fail exams' you are setting the scene for exactly that to happen. You would never make such a harsh statement to a friend. Rather, you would provide positive, encouraging, and optimistic counsel to them. You would be objective, mindful of the facts, and would not incite hysteria. You would give them positive feedback about how they are working, reminding them of what they have already achieved to date. Do the same for yourself. Help yourself. Positive visualization will help; imagine yourself turning over an exam paper and seeing questions to which you know the answers, feel your anxiety dissipate as you realize you can do this. Now turn that thought into reality.

Visualization

Visualization is also known as 'playing the movie to the end'. Pressing fast forward and looking ahead to see how the choices you make today impact upon the future. In the short term, imagine the day after the exam, when you receive your results. Visualize yourself in your workplace and think about yourself smiling, nodding, receiving congratulations, basking in the glory as you confirm that, yes indeed, you did pass. Watch the secretary put an announcement on the department noticeboard. Now compare that situation to one where you have failed. Commiserations instead of congratulations, the dread of meeting consultants who are full of expectation with their raised eyebrows. Imagine the awkwardness when those who do not know ask, time and time again, 'How did you get on in London?'

Think of this moment. Think of which outcome you want and about what you can do today to help make it happen.

Pass first time

The period of studying required to obtain adequate knowledge across the breadth of the curriculum takes up a lot of time, a period of several months, and entails significant opportunity costs. In an effort to minimize disruption to life as you know it, aim to do each exam once only, and do each of them right first time. The first attempt at doing anything is the one most likely to succeed. This is when motivation and self belief are highest and the thought of failure has not yet occurred. Put 100% effort into your preparation the first sitting: do not slack, do not be too lenient with yourself, and you will not prolong the misery by having to take exams a second time.

Figure 2.1 shows how motivation is high at the beginning of exam preparation but is maintained at this level only for a limited period of time before it begins to decrease at point X. Motivation reduces continually as time continues to pass. It is important to maximize your early efforts; motivation gets you started but you must form a study habit to prolong your campaign. Good habits will keep you studying long enough to pass the exam before the decline in motivation can be compounded by failure at the initial attempt.

It is important to get everything in place to help you succeed, as shown in Figure 2.2. Just as for intubation—when success is dependent upon positioning, the correct equipment, and assistance—all must be primed and ready to help you when required. While timing and concentration are also important factors for intubation, these same rules apply to exam preparation. You need to be able to focus to study effectively. You need time, you need space, and you need help. You may need a nanny or a granny to help with children. You will need space in your head to focus and should clear your mind by delegating other tasks or paying someone else to do them. The temporary expense of a cleaner, a gardener, or having your supermarket shopping delivered will be worth every penny by allowing you to study uninterrupted. You will need the support of friends and family who understand why you are less available to them and you should be honest about the level of commitment these exams require. You need the will to succeed. It is a tiring time and mood is often low. An element of pastoral support and empathy from all

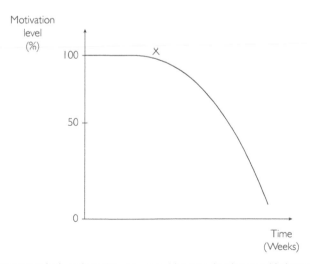

Figure 2.1 Motivation is high early in the campaign. Use it to develop good habits which will last throughout.

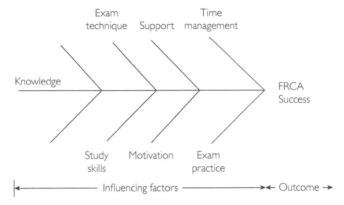

Figure 2.2 Fish-bone diagram: factors influencing exam outcome.

quarters helps more than a 'I did it when it was much harder while working 167 hours per week' approach. Support from others taking the exam or who have recently passed it will be helpful for studying and empathy. Do not be afraid to ask for help.

Similarly, in anaesthesia, the first attempt is when the likelihood of success is greatest, be it for intubation, inserting an arterial line, or siting an epidural. Each subsequent attempt is less likely to be successful (although the cumulative chance of success increases slightly each time). We have all struggled and struggled to find the epidural space, only to ask a colleague for help and watch them drop it in effortlessly at the first attempt. Was it easier for them? Are they just better at epidurals? Not necessarily. It is because our colleague was on their first attempt, with all its inherent advantages, whereas we (you) have sunk into the mindset of 'Can't do it. Got to do it. Have not managed to do it this time either. Don't think I'll ever get it in' and are spiralling rapidly downwards in a vicious circle. We did not think like this before our first attempt, our confidence was high then, but now, at subsequent attempts, we have lost faith in our ability to succeed.

Having confidence in your ability *does* influence the outcome. If you watch a medical student attempting to site an intravenous cannula, they can be seen shaking their head as they first look at the vein. The needle is barely through the skin before they announce it is not in and request swabs and the sharps box. You *know* they were never going to be successful because they did not believe they could be successful, and this became a self-fulfilling prophecy.

This is exactly what happens when trainees fail their exam. They become despondent at the thought of all the work they have done and the time they have spent studying, and feel it was all for nothing, time wasted. They also have to subject themselves to several more months of the same studying and sacrifices, all while dealing with the mental attitude of 'I'm never going to pass'. The longer this continues, the worse it gets and the more insurmountable the exams become.

In order to avoid this situation occurring, plan to pass the exam at the first attempt. Easier said than done I hear you say, and perhaps rightly so, but you must, *must* make your first attempt a good attempt, while your motivation is high.

Make a good attempt

Anyone can have a bad day at the exam, but to fail while knowing you did not put in the effort beforehand to do yourself justice will be far worse.

What do I mean by a good attempt? Firstly, I mean do not 'have a go' at the exam. If you have a go to 'see if you can get it' you are very unlikely to do so. Passing the FRCA is not a chance phenomenon; it is the result of a long period of focussed study and learning.

Secondly, put some effort into actively making this first attempt the best it can be. Have everything set up in a way that will maximize your chance of early success. For comparison, imagine you are going to site an epidural in an obese parturient. You would never merely expose the back, insert the needle, and begin advancing it in the hope you may just stumble across the epidural space. If you did, you would be unlikely to succeed and may cause significant harm. Instead, you would recognize this as a challenging procedure and plan accordingly. You plan ahead, pay attention to details, and have everything in place to help you, before you begin. You may ask an assistant to help with positioning. You will assess the back and identify the midline carefully before deciding where to insert your needle. Apply the same care and attention to your exam preparation. Plan your studying in advance, think about how long you need to cover the curriculum. Identify the hurdles and decide how you will surmount them. Identify the threats to success and how you will minimize them. Plan to start studying six months before the exam date and progress to doing little other than studying in the final three months. Studying more frequently for shorter periods will place you a long way down the road to success. Cramming for the FRCA does not work: it makes you tired, unable to concentrate, inefficient, ineffective, and panicked. Remember, you are the rule, not the exception to it. No half-hearted attempts at high-stakes exams.

Timing

When is the right time to sit the exam? Sitting the final FRCA too early shows up candidates with less clinical experience; they do not sound convincing nor do they portray clinical confidence in their decision making. Sitting the exam too late risks delaying progression to higher and advanced training, as all components of the exam must be passed by the end of the ST4 (specialty training) year. At the time of writing, this is under review by the Royal College of Anaesthetists (RCoA).

In basic training, there is very little time to gain all components of the Primary FRCA as all parts are required prior to application for ST3 training (as the rules stand at the time of writing). Too early is difficult, as there is so much that is new in CT1 (core training) and you are, quite correctly, focussed on the Initial Assessment of Competency (IAC) and learning about anaesthetic drugs and the anaesthetic machine at first.

There will never be a perfect time to sit the exams, so you should not wait for it to present itself. It is easier to be selfish with your time if you are single and live alone. Having no one to think about but yourself allows for greater immersion into exam preparation and fewer considerations to prioritize. But this option has long passed for many. To postpone having children until the exams are passed is a luxury few have. Starting or expanding a family is an important consideration for both women and men; aside from the anecdotal disadvantage of 'baby brain' and hormonal lability, a prolonged period of disturbed nights for either partner is not conducive to studying effectively. However, postponing the exam until your child reaches a specific milestone will not necessarily avoid disruption. Each stage of child development brings its own unique set of patterns and routines (or lack thereof), and the challenge to both partners will continue.

It makes sense, however, to plan when to sit the exam as best you can. You need to allow six months for preparation, the final three being particularly intense. Postpone your exam sitting if your wedding and honeymoon occur during this period but, otherwise, do not delay.

Define your motivation

The usual reason for doing postgraduate exams is for career progression. In anaesthesia, trainees cannot progress to higher and advanced training, and then to a consultant post, without the final FRCA exam. The ultimate goal of most, but not all, trainees entering specialist training is to complete the training programme and gain a CCT in anaesthesia. Post Fellowship, colleagues now know you are the 'real deal', and will extend to you a healthy amount of respect, befitting of someone who has accomplished the accolade of FRCA. It is not an easy exam and many good anaesthetists do not pass. With the FRCA in hand, you are now on the home straight to becoming a consultant and existing consultants will begin to view you as a potential consultant colleague.

The exams of the RCoA are arguably among the hardest to pass. This is a good thing; ensuring a high standard of clinical practice and patient safety, and keeping the profession held in high regard. However, not all trainees will pass and some may decide against repeated attempts and avoid the incumbent stress. At some levels of training, there is an option to rescind your training number and move sidewards to become a specialty doctor. The roles and responsibility of being a consultant are not for everyone, and many have long and rewarding careers in these alternative posts. There are advantages to this move which may suit some doctors. It removes the time pressure of the training clock, the working patterns are different, and the goals are individual. If you *really* do not want to study or take exams (or have tried and failed), then this may be an attractive option for you. However, you should consider this carefully as a return to training from these posts is not common and the pass rate of specialty doctors in exams is lower than that of doctors in training posts.

Assuming that if you are still reading, you do wish to take these exams, it is then a matter of finding the bucketful of motivation you need to get on with studying.

What is your motivation? Why do you want to pass the exam? Think hard about this because you must *really* want it to make the sacrifices required. I have been impressed by the determination and tenacity I have seen in several doctors—doctors in non-consultant career grades taking these exams time and time again, becoming more determined to pass each time and never giving up. I have known doctors from overseas who are adamant they will not leave the UK without FRCA after their name. They often take multiple attempts at exams at huge personal cost, both financial and otherwise, but such is their motivation to achieve this prestigious qualification, they usually succeed in the end. The lesson? You must really want to pass and you should not give up.

For adult learners, motivation must come from within and learning must be self-directed, goal-orientated, and perceived as clinically relevant. Didactic teaching is not required; adults do not need to be taught facts. The factual knowledge comprising the exam syllabus is clearly stated in the 2010 Curriculum and, by this age and stage, each candidate can find this information from their preferred resource. Adults need to *discover* the answers to their questions and find the relevance of them to their clinical work. Problems getting to grips with basic physics is common in the final FRCA. At this stage, you know how to use equipment but do not have the principles underpinning its mechanism at the forefront of your mind—a bit like driving a car. However, with a car, you do not set off unless it is working correctly, whereas we do need to anaesthetize patients when they are ill. We need to understand the equipment we use so we can troubleshoot problems. Teaching new start anaesthetists or explaining to medical students in theatre about breathing systems and gas flow is a good way to ensure you revisit the important principles of equipment regularly, until they become ingrained in your mind.

As adults, teachers, and learners become more equal. Both are mature professionals, and the usual age difference between the two is often not significant. As adult learners we need help to develop automatic routines for conveying knowledge in the correct format for the exam and to propagate studying by maintaining motivation in the lead up to the exam. As children, we were motivated by peer pressure, ranking in the class, and fear of parental disappointment. As adults, it is different. Our lives are no longer purely for school, learning, and preparing for exams. We no longer have weeks off to cram beforehand and any leave we do take is usually earmarked for a well-earned holiday; we are loathe to spend it studying. We no longer live in fear of our report card nor do we get rewards from our parents for good exam grades.

I hear trainees say 'I'm no good at exams' and 'I always fail physiology', but others 'always pass anyway'. One theory gaining popularity is that there is no such thing as natural talent; it all boils down to hard work and putting in the hours. Those perceived to have natural talent (the Williams sisters, Tiger Woods) have been learning their craft since they were toddlers. They have prac-tised six days per week, every week. They have spent hours playing the sport and more hours attaining the associated fitness and mental targets.

Tell yourself you are good at exams. Look how far you have come compared to the general population, compared to non-medical friends perhaps, or compared to when you were a new start in anaesthesia. Believing you have the ability to pass will go a long way in helping you to ac-tually succeed. Successful sportspeople work hard with psychologists until they believe they can win. Alternatively, identify a particularly poor role model in your department (if there is one) and make note that they managed to pass these exams. If they can do it, anyone can do it and most certainly, you can do it.

Motivation to work hard in the short term is difficult when the rewards are only apparent in the long term. This is true for many lifestyle changes. Losing weight is all short-term deprivation for results only apparent in the long term. Giving up smoking causes acute withdrawal symptoms and cravings, with health benefits promised years ahead. Anything worth having will not come easily.

If you spend three hours per day, every day, studying for the exam, you will become expert in that discipline. Can you put in three hours per day? Every day? The amount of effort you are prepared to put in and the sacrifices you are prepared to make depend on how much you want the result. In 2013, Scottish tennis player Andy Murray did not return to the UK to be presented with the Sports Personality of the Year award as it took place shortly before the Australian Open and would have interrupted his training programme and rehabilitation schedule in the USA. That shows a long-term commitment to win, and one that he did not want to jeopardize by short-term thrills.

Your short-term thrills (the pub, your family, your friends on Facebook) will still be waiting for you after the exam. Prioritize yourself and this exam for now. Write down five things that you waste time over. When do you do these activities? Now write down times of the day and days of the week that you could re-allocate for studying. Your two lists may not be exactly the same but if you ensure there is significant overlap between the two, you can fit studying into as much 'wasted' time as possible and perhaps leave some of the more enjoyable parts of your week in-tact. However, if this is not possible, do not give up what you want most, for what you want now.

Incentivization

Incentives to study will provide short- and medium-term goals while you work towards your long-term goal of exam success. You should make goals which are specific, time-based, realistic, and achievable. Make several at a time so that there are always a variety of objectives to aim for and which answer the inevitable question of 'What's the point?'. You could plan a holiday after the exam, or if annual leave is in short supply, book a spa day at a local health retreat. If you study tonight from 6 p.m. to 9 p.m., you can watch television afterwards or meet friends who went to the pub earlier. If money motivates you, put the money you save from your reduced social life aside each week and use it to treat yourself to something extravagant after the exam. Short-term goals include studying for 45 minutes before watching television for a short time, or rewarding a 30-minute period of work with coffee and a biscuit. Focussing on small steps and rewarding each one when completed will keep you motivated to continue and help avoid that overwhelming feel-ing of there being so much still to do that you will never get it all done (so why bother starting?). Medium-term objectives such as studying each weekday night to allow a night off to relax on Sat-urday will keep your motivation up throughout the week.

All this is important because your goal is to pass first time. Do not forget that your first at-tempt at any exam is the one that has most chance of success. Therefore, you must ensure it is a good attempt.

CHAPTER 3

Time management

You will never find time for anything. If you want time you must make it.
Charles Buxton (1875–1942, English Philanthropist)

CONTENTS

You need time to study. Extra time cannot be made; instead it must be carved out of that we already have . . . or words to that effect. Within a week, there are 168 hours. Taking into account full-time employment (48 hours), this leaves 120 hours. Allowing eight hours of sleep per day (particularly important when studying) will leave 64 hours per week (or over nine hours per day) available for studying and leisure. I suggest to potential exam candidates that they aim to spend three hours per day studying during the final three months leading up to the exam, regardless of what they have done beforehand. At first glance, this looks to be eminently possible and still leaves six hours of free time per day. When you examine your week closely and decide where you will fit studying in, you will undoubtedly identify periods of wasted time, which you can then harness and use to better effect. Identify and write down these periods of time now, if you have not already done so.

Discipline and saboteurs

In order to sustain any study regime, self-discipline is required. Often the hardest part is just getting started. If you find yourself filing your nails, sharpening your pencils, or cleaning the grout in the bathroom with an old toothbrush, you are not being disciplined enough and are sabotaging your own plans. Go back and reread Chapter 2 on motivation and decide if and why you really want to pass this exam. Next, write down what you were doing during each of the last 24 hours. This will help you to see the periods of time which could be put to better use.

It is best to establish a routine for studying. Decide where it best fits into each day and try to be consistent about studying in this time. Motivation gets you started but habit will keep you going when motivation declines with time. Good habits can be made as easily as bad habits and establishing a set routine for studying will avoid having to make a daily decision to make it happen: it will happen automatically, becoming just what you do at that designated time.

During this designated period of time, a multitude of time saboteurs must be actively managed as lost time is never found again. Many are simple: stop playing with your mobile phone, stop surfing aimlessly on the internet (enjoyable though this may be), avoid social media, do not watch television indiscriminately. Record your favourite television programmes and watch them when you are resting after a night shift or when you achieve your study goals and are rewarded with television time. Do not study with an internet connection close at hand; you *will* get distracted and find yourself 'just checking this' or 'just doing that'. Do not kid yourself you need it for studying. You will be tempted to google every idea that pops into your head and, once started, we always spend more time online than originally intended. It is useful to make a quick note of things that occur to you that you do need to remember to do later. Once down on the list, you can put them aside, mentally as well as physically. They are removed from your mind, leaving you free to concentrate entirely on the subject matter and able to relax now you know you will not forget them.

Wasting small amounts of time will add up and you will either achieve very little in your three hours or you will be sitting at your desk for a lot longer than necessary. (Note, however, that being at your desk does not equate with studying.) Both outcomes will annoy you and make you feel disinclined to study the next time. Telephone calls, home administration, cooking, texting—to name but a few alternative pursuits—can all wait until your three hours of studying is complete. At the end of the three hours ask yourself what you have learned? This question will show you if you have been studying effectively or not. If you cannot recall what you have learned, you need to go back, revisit it, repeat it until you can remember it. I am sorry to say that there are no shortcuts.

Self-discipline is easier if you are interested in what you are studying. Choose to study something you saw at work that day or the knowledge competencies relevant to cases you managed during your last time on call. Change topic within the three hours. Move from subject to subject (just as in the viva), keeping your brain active and your mind engaged. Change your mode of learning: swap reading for writing, or books for flash cards. Make changes as often as necessary to keep boredom at bay and decide when (and if) to factor in a tea break.

Delegation

Several commitments at home can be delegated. If having a messy or unclean home irritates you to the point of being unable to let it be, hire a cleaner or ask your housemates to take on your duties. If there never seems to be food in the fridge, organize a home delivery and avoid repeated trips to the supermarket or eating take-away food each night. Arrange to have your milk delivered, your shirts ironed, your windows cleaned—do anything you can identify as being helpful to you and achieving your goal. Again, put these costs in the context of the time and money you will spend resitting the exam if you do not make this attempt as good as possible.

Spending time wisely

Time spent on leisure activities must be carefully considered in terms of opportunity cost. You may need to miss trips to the cinema or the shopping centre; you may decide you cannot afford to spend an hour on the telephone talking to your mum, at the expense of studying. Sacrifices do need to be made, and you should not give up what you want in the long term for what you want right now. Remember all these changes need only be for a short while. If you apply maximum effort and pass first time, you will find that shops, films, novels, restaurants, and gyms will still be there and you will then have copious amounts of free time to enjoy spending as you wish.

As mentioned earlier, it is easier to sit and pass exams when the only individual to consider is yourself and all your time is your own. However, by this stage in life, it is common to have a significant other and/or children. Partners must be made aware of the importance of studying for and passing these exams, and also need reminding that these hardships are only for a finite period. Hopefully, with explanation, they will be understanding of your priorities. Evenings in front of the television, casual nights out to the pub, impromptu trips out for dinner need to take second place to fitting in the three hours of studying each day. It may be possible to pacify some with a simultaneous subscription to Sky Sports or Sky Movies while you are otherwise engaged, and this will again be money well spent.

Children and childcare are less straightforward. The big issue for many at this stage is balancing work with childcare and spending time with their children. There is no good time in your child's life for mummy or daddy to be studying and sitting exams, so best it has to happen once only. Whether you have newborns not yet sleeping well, babies weaning, toddlers teething, or a child starting nursery, school, or university, there will always be difficult transitions to deal with. It is not worth postponing the exam on these grounds, as you could find yourself doing this indefinitely. Particularly for those training full-time, the training clock is ticking and the exam window is limited.

If you have childcare provision, consider paying (or asking) for an extra session or an extra day to allow you to devote your attention to studying. Far from missing your child, it may make the time you spend with them more meaningful and special. Your child will be none the wiser if they are very small and will not remember if they are less than four years old. (Older than this, you can explain it to them.) Again, put the cost of childcare in context. Similarly, if you can request a favour from grandparents to take the children for a weekend, do so, but instead of a having a wild night out and a long lie in, hit the books, bank some study time, and enjoy some uninterrupted sleep. Have friends take your kids for play dates. It is not forever and you will be able to return the favour in due course. If these options are too drastic, ask your partner, friends, or relatives to take the children out of your way for an afternoon, and do not waste a moment of the time alone.

Many candidates state they would do 'anything' to pass the exam. If this is truly the case, prioritizing yourself and your own needs above those of others in your life is one of the best things you can do to help yourself. Decide what this means you must do in your own life.

I am not suggesting you can do nothing but study during the three months leading up to the exam; rather, that leisure time and activities need to carefully considered and prioritized appropriately. The efficient way to cope with demands on your time is to compartmentalize it into clearly defined studying time and leisure time. Studying effectively for one hour, then having an hour of leisure time, is much better than a half-hearted effort at studying for two hours. After dinner, you can choose to devote yourself to the children's bath and bedtime routine or the evening news between 6 p.m. and 7 p.m., leaving you time to study from 7 p.m. to 10 p.m. and to relax from 10 p.m. until 11 p.m. Or you may prefer to study from 6 p.m. until 9 p.m. and watch television or surf the net a bit later. You can study all day Saturday and play golf on Sunday. Or you can study Saturday and Sunday mornings and have the afternoons off. The point is that you have to get the study time in each day, then assess how much remaining time there is to spend on other pursuits.

Getting started

Getting started is one of the hardest parts of studying but, once under way, it is never as bad as expected. Whether it is starting the whole project six months in advance (yes, six months is what you should be planning) or getting down to today's planned subjects, the biggest threat to time management is procrastination. We are all guilty of this and it varies from having another cup of coffee and a chat before you start, to making an elaborately colour-coded, beautifully highlighted study plan. There is no point sitting at your desk doing a quick suduko or texting or whatever you are prone to doing when seeking to put something off. These do not count as studying but waste your studying time. Try the five-minute rule: tell yourself you will do five minutes of studying before reassessing how you feel. Do you still feel unable to do it? Can you remember why you wanted to pass this exam? Usually, things will be fine once you are started, and you will continue, but if you are truly not in a frame of mind conducive to studying, cut your losses and have the night off. Far better to enjoy some proper free time and relax rather than sit glumly at your desk for the allotted time yet achieve nothing. Bear in mind, however, that you cannot do this each and every time you sit down! You may have to give yourself a 'tough love' type of pep talk. After all, whatever else happens, you have to do the work yourself, if you are to pass the exam.

Procrastination is not the sign of laziness or dithering, as many believe it to be. What it signals is a fear of failure at some level, and this makes us reluctant to begin doing that which we perceive as being difficult. It is much easier to practise multiple-choice questions (MCQs) from a book than it is to go back to basics and learn the principles of how the ultrasound scanner works. The latter is a much better use of time but unknown topics induce fear and reluctance in all of us. Instead of hoping the subjects which cause you most difficulty will not appear in the exams, be proactive, assume they will be asked, learn about them inside out, and turn them from being your most dreaded topics into small gifts from the examiner! Try doing this instead of taking a 'head in the sand' approach. Do not be victim to the question bank! Prepare in advance, in this way. Do not passively wait until the day of the exam, then wish you had done more work. In fact, if a topic is springing to mind as you read this, put this book down and go and learn about that topic now.

Procrastination makes your goal of exam success even harder to achieve by robbing you of precious studying time. Do not let this happen to you. Recognize procrastination and eliminate it.

Working hours

It is tempting to assign your time spent at work in the hospital as being just that—time for work in which no studying is possible. Particularly when on call, it is tempting, when quiet, to watch television or read magazines. You justify this slack time to yourself by thinking 'If I was busy, I wouldn't be able to study anyway'. This is true, but if you are not busy, you can choose to either capitalize on it by studying during time that is not your 'own' anyway, or you must assign it to the 'relaxation time' compartment and acknowledge you are partaking of it now, while on call, rather than at some point in the future. Relaxation time is precious and is more enjoyable spent outside the hospital, in comfortable surroundings, with company of your choosing. Do not waste time hanging around chatting at work when you could be doing something more useful instead.

Daytime work commitments are huge learning opportunities if you choose to make the most of them. Do not think it is 'just another day on Intensive Care'. Set relevant objectives to achieve during the day: nutritional requirements of a particular patient, for example. Speak to the dietitian about the required components of enteral feed and total parenteral nutrition (TPN). How are they calculated? Talk to the pharmacist about how such a feed is prepared and to the nurses on the practicalities of giving it. Do not sit trying to learn a table full of grams of nitrogen and numbers of calories (although you may need to know some of these, too). By putting the information into a clinical context, and remembering the TPN you prescribed for Mr X or Mrs Y, it will become much more memorable. If you are ever asked about nutritional requirements of the critically ill or malnourishment in the elderly, you will immediately think of these patients and their associated problems and treatments.

During a theatre list (for example, Ear, Nose, and Throat–ENT), ask your consultant why they chose the technique they did. Have they always done it this way? How else could it be done and what are the advantages of each way? What do other ENT anaesthetists in your department do for a case like this or that? What are the current thoughts on best practice? What needs consideration at a practical level? How could this be asked about in the exam? Anaesthetic nurses or Operating Department Practitioners (ODPs) are full of information and will be able to tell you the usual practices of many colleagues.

Learning in theatre about a topic relevant to the patient contextualizes knowledge and makes it easier to recall. Observing how falling oxygen saturations on one lung are managed when the chest is opened, makes a bigger impression than reading the chapter in the book on ventilation perfusion mismatching during thoracic surgery. I cannot stress enough that it is much easier to learn and remember from a day at work compared to merely reading a textbook. During a long bowel operation, learn the definition of enhanced recovery. What does it consist of? Find out how the cardiac output monitor you are using actually works and what other types are available. Read about nerve blocks before your orthopaedic list. Ask your consultant to quiz you on the anatomy the next day or to clarify any unclear areas. In theatre, you can revise intrathecal opioids, causes of deep vein thromboses (DVTs), cooling and hypothermia, cell salvage and transfusion, and so on.

Make every case or list you do an opportunity upon which to hang the relevant knowledge competencies. When the theatre day is over, read about the things you have seen and consolidate any new points you have learned, perhaps augmenting it with some textbook work. This revisiting, building upon, and reinforcing of prior knowledge is called 'spiral learning' and it is very effective. You will be able to tick off several core clinical learning outcomes (CCLOs) stated in annexes B and C of the RCoA 2010 curriculum, all within a day's work. How productive will you feel going home that evening? You will also feel enthused about your continued learning, have reinforced your self-belief, and begin to sense that this exam really is achievable.

Clinical experience

The same rationale applies to the advice to arrange taster days. The exam closely follows the 2010 Curriculum. All areas of this will be sampled over the course of all components of the exam. Gaps in knowledge due to lack of experience are common in the final FRCA written exam and are noticeable in the structured oral exam (SOE) element. There is currently a recommendation in the Chairman's report that taster days should be arranged in sub-specialty training units of which the candidate has no experience prior to the final FRCA. If you have not seen a cardiac bypass circuit or a craniotomy, have never been to a chronic pain clinic or theatre session, take some time to go, prior to the exam. Again, it is much easier to remember what to do and how to do it if you have seen a case where those things happened; it provides you with a context in which to house your knowledge.

Make contact and arrange to spend a day in specific theatres. You need to be proactive about such things and should contact the college tutor or department secretary in the first instance. The agreement of these specialist departments is required to accommodate the needs of exam candidates as well as their current trainees, and you should ensure this practice is supported by the training committee in your school. You may need to take a day of annual leave or attend during days off work following night or weekend shifts. This counts as your studying time and not working hours. This is the way you are choosing to learn about a new topic. It is not extra work, nor is it unpaid work, nor will it cause you to breach the European Working Time Directive (EWTD) ruling about number of hours worked. You will be there in an entirely supernumerary capacity, solely to see and learn.

This approach to seeking out additional training is not only useful for specialist units of training. If there are gaps in your logbook, there will be gaps in your clinical experience and gaps in your exam knowledge. Identify these early and ensure you spend a day, at least, in such theatres in your own hospital, to gain experience in that particular field of anaesthesia. You can do this outwith your normal hours of work. Again, it does not count as work. Being in theatre is how you are choosing to study this subject on this day.

Make use of opportunities that crop up: if your day happens to finish earlier than expected, use the time available to join another theatre and see something else. Relate each case you see to a topic on your list of things to cover. Maximizing your clinical experience is the best way to remember and understand the facts you need to know. Going home early 'to study' will lead to coffee and procrastination until dinner time and you will have nothing to show for your early finish.

Your time is yours to manage. Treat it like the precious commodity it is and use it wisely.

CHAPTER 4

Study skills

Tell me and I forget. Teach me and I remember. Involve me and I learn.

Benjamin Franklin

CONTENTS

Having found time in your day to study, you must now use it effectively. In this chapter, we will look at some ways to make your studying more effective. There are three main types of learner recognized: visual learners, auditory learners, and kinaesthetic learners. These categories are self-explanatory and are evident in all fields of teaching and learning. As very young children, we are all kinaesthetic learners who learn about the surrounding world by touching, feeling, doing, and becoming involved. As we mature, we develop the skills of visual learning and auditory learning, to varying degrees. In reality, we are each a mixture of all three types but will have one method that predominates, and that method is how we learn best. Identifying where your strengths lie will enable you to utilize a method of studying which will be most effective.

Accessible aids

Try to have different study aids available and easily accessible at all times. If your books and notes are neatly packed away upstairs in a high cupboard in the study at the far end of the house, it will require significant effort to get to them, get them out, and begin using them. For small periods of time, it will hardly seem worth the bother. So you will not bother. This inertia can be avoided by having books littered around the lounge or kitchen, next to your laptop—wherever you spend significant amounts of time.

Being messy during exam preparation should be better tolerated by those around you and you may well be forgiven for this finite period. By always having something close at hand, you will be able to make use of every spare five minutes here and there. You could cover one CCLO, at least, in five minutes. All those five-minute intervals will soon add up and you will have created some useful study time from what is normally dead time in your day.

Learning occurs best when studying is regular and frequent. At work, have some form of learning material in your bag, in your locker, or in the department. You will quickly become able to study in a variety of environments; like every skill, studying improves the more often it is practised, and your studying will become efficient and effective if you practice it often. Short periods of study will also help you to get started more quickly during your longer sessions and you will avoid the tendency to have a coffee, check your emails, or catch up with the ironing before getting started on the task in hand.

Use the gaps between patients to revise the pharmacology of the drugs and fluids you plan to use for the next case. This way you will read about drugs used frequently more often than drugs used rarely. If you administer and read about fentanyl six times throughout a shift, you will be able to recall the half life and plasma protein binding values quickly. Remember, drugs are the tools of our trade and there is no excuse for not knowing everything about a drug you routinely administer to patients, both in the exam and in clinical practice. During a routine case, when the patient is stable, challenge yourself to reproduce graphs or diagrams pertinent to the exam: a schematic of the epidural space or the brachial plexus, a normal spirometry tracing, an abnormal capnograph trace, or the three graphs determining cerebral perfusion and oxygenation. At all times remember diagrams should be large, clear, neat, have straight lines, with axes labelled with the units of measurement; tables should have a title; and anatomical drawings need to show their orientation. The overall look should resemble the London Underground map more closely than Spaghetti Junction.

Make your own luck

Some people get lucky in exams. The questions to which they know the answers just seem to appear at each exam. Others are unlucky and get asked all the difficult questions on topics that, as they freely admit, they would never have studied in a million years. The lucky ones have studied thoroughly and will know the answers to nearly any question which may come up. The unlucky ones have gaps in their knowledge. The more you prepare, the luckier you will become.

Write down the five topics which you would least like to meet in your exam. Actually write them down now. When you have done this, put this list somewhere you can see it often. Keep it there until you have learned these five topics well enough to be able to answer them confidently. Then, repeat the exercise with your next five least desirable topics. You will make your own luck by identifying the topics you find most difficult; becoming knowledgeable about difficult subject areas is a much better strategy than adopting a 'head in the sand' approach. Familiarity with topics you find difficult will reduce anxiety and improve performance. Make sure that the first time you consider the route of the trigeminal nerve is not when you are at the viva exam. Use this technique successfully and you will never fear an exam question again.

There are opposing theories about the factors which are important in determining whether or not an individual will become successful in any field. One school of thought believes that success occurs through a series of serendipitous events: when you were born, your physique, your parents' careers, their outlook on life, all helped along by a hefty portion of luck. This school think much of the pathway in life is predetermined and lucky individuals need only take advantage of the opportunities that spontaneously come their way. Others may be equally as intelligent but lack the same infrastructure around them and will never reach the same heights of success. The other school of thought is that we each get out what we put in, and through hard work can achieve our maximum potential regardless of external factors, if our will is great enough. There is a belief that 10,000 hours of practice is required to achieve mastery of any subject, be it piano playing or golf.

No matter which theory you believe, if you want to pass the exam you need to study, and study hard. We will discuss what studying hard means both in terms of time and efficacy, shortly.

Break down the syllabus

The exam syllabus comprises the knowledge components of the 2010 Curriculum. To cover the curriculum is a large task. It seems a huge amount to get through, and indeed it *is* a huge amount to get through. It can be overwhelming and leave one wondering where to start. Too much fear and anxiety can have a paralyzing effect which will not help. Avoid becoming overwhelmed by the enormity of the whole task. Even breaking it down into units of training—cardiac anaesthesia, chronic pain, and so on—still leaves large topics to be tackled. You must break these units down further to define the required knowledge components and arrange them into small manageable groups to be tackled one by one. Appendices B and C of the curriculum does this for you. Cardiothoracic anaesthesia has 24 CCLOs including 'Understands rational behind warming and cooling patients and the complications that this may cause' and 'Can describe the anaesthetic considerations associated with "off-pump" surgery'. These bite-sized units of revision can be addressed in turn. When you have little time available, you may cover only one. At times when you cannot motivate yourself to begin studying, you could aim to do only one such objective and then reassess your situation. Anything more than this is a bonus. The chances are that once started, you will be able to keep going.

To save having to refer to Appendices B and C online each time, I suggest you print off these lengthy documents and then cut them up into strips, with two or three competencies on each piece of paper. The resultant pile is your syllabus. Take one or two to work each day; pick three or four to cover in a study session. You could even have a lucky dip! Enjoy watching the pile of paper diminish as the exam date approaches.

Target the past papers

All previous short answer question (SAQ) papers are published on the website of the RCoA to aid candidates in their exam revision. Use them—but use them properly. Do not simply glance over them thinking 'Yep, could do that' or 'That one's a bit tricky, hope that doesn't come up'. There is no value in that approach and you will not learn simply by osmosis from reading the answer plans. Instead, you must choose one question at a time. Sit down and allocate yourself 12 minutes and actually **write the answer down** as you would in the exam. This way you can see what you know, you practise conveying it, and you will identify gaps in your knowledge, which in turn means you can correct them. They are now 'known unknowns'.

You may find you know lots and lots about a subject, so much so that you cannot extract the important points efficiently in the 12 minutes allowed. Remember, there are no extra marks for extra knowledge. You must not spend more time than allowed on any one question as this will be to the detriment of others as well as to your overall score. Even the well-prepared, knowledgeable candidate needs to practise accessing and presenting their knowledge optimally in the exam format. Make sure that the first time you try is always a practice; do not leave it until the exam day to find out that you cannot decide how best to lay out your answer or to wonder if a table format might have worked better. You can even give your written script to someone else and see how legible or otherwise they find your writing. Twelve minutes is not a long time and little pockets of time can be found among an evening filled with television, adverts, and waiting for the kettle to boil.

Why only 12 minutes? Twelve questions in three hours allows 15 minutes per question. However, 15 minutes is an absolute maximum and, if used entirely, will allow no time for reading the paper over at the start, moving between questions, and filling in gaps at the end. All SAQ questions can be answered within 10 minutes, using one side of A4 paper. Running out of time is a common complaint from candidates about this paper and you must learn to be disciplined. In the West of Scotland School of Anaesthesia, we have trialled exam practice allowing both 12 and 15 minutes per question. When the time allowed was increased to 15 minutes, candidates still ran out of time. With continual practice at 12 minutes per question, candidates reported that they had plenty of time in the exam and felt calmed by knowing they were not behind schedule.

Examples of MCQs are widely available but are of variable quality. The questions released by the RCoA are the best markers of the standard required. It goes without saying that you should use all of the exam resources available on the RCoA website including past questions and videos of good and bad performances in a Structured Oral Examination (SOE). 'E-learning Anaesthesia' is another good source of exam-standard questions (available at http://www.rcoa.ac.uk/e-la).

Single best answers (SBAs) are newer, having only been introduced to the FRCA in September 2011. The bank of questions is therefore smaller and, as these questions are more difficult to produce, many fewer are released for practice. This situation should improve with time.

Chairman's report

The Chairman of Exams produces a report after each sitting of the written SAQ paper. It is available on the RCoA website (under exam resources) and you should read it. It is a gold-mine of information. Look for clues in the report. There are often comments such as 'This question was answered badly by many candidates' or 'Fewer than 50% of candidates passed this question' or 'This question was a good discriminator' (that is to say, those who passed the question, passed the paper overall). These comments indicate questions that are most likely to be repeated in a subsequent paper, particularly those questions asking about basic topics, such as oxygen and pre-oxygenation, or common occurrences such as massive obstetric haemorrhage. The exams schedule is such that questions cannot be repeated in the subsequent paper, so it is usually at least a year before they can appear again.

What about new techniques and topical or contentious issues? There is a point past which a new drug, technique, or guideline changes from occasional or selective use by only a few, and therefore deemed too new for the exam, to becoming accepted practice for all and a suitable mainstream topic to include. Publications which inform changes to practice filter slowly through the cohort of practitioners, who take them up at different rates. Not until they become accepted common practice will they appear in the exam. However, remember that what is deemed too new for the SAQ paper may be perfectly in time for the SOE eight to ten months later.

The current trend in the final FRCA is to include questions pertaining to published national guidelines relevant to the curriculum, as well as information published from bodies such as the General Medical Council (GMC). Educational supplements to the *British Journal of Anaesthesia* (*BJA*) may also give rise to questions. What were the last guidelines produced by the National Institute for Health and Care Excellence (NICE), or the World Health Organization (WHO)? What about patient safety groups? What was the most recent 'glossy' produced by the Association of Anaesthetists of Great Britain and Ireland (AAGBI)? These will cover current issues and are likely to crop up in one part of the exam or another. Make sure you have read them and understand the key messages within.

MCQ practice

There are many books and DVDs available to practise MCQ technique. These are of variable quality and not all of them reflect the standard of the actual exam. This way of learning is good in some respects. It is good for practising reading the questions accurately, for working within a time frame, and for gauging your level of knowledge by scoring your answers. It is not, however, a good primary means of gaining and retaining knowledge. For example, if you score poorly on a question comparing fentanyl and alfentanil, it is much better to go back to a pharmacology textbook and learn about each drug in its entirety, rather than gleaning isolated and unrelated facts from the answer page. Not only are these facts difficult to remember and recall in isolation, but there are many similar but different questions over which you can easily confuse yourself if your knowledge is not sound and does not come from basic principles.

Once you have learned about each drug independent of others, you can compare their pharmacokinetics, and relate those variables to what you know of each drug from clinical use. MCQs ask sporadic questions and, while studying, you should complement practice questions with a more holistic view of the topic.

'Proper' studying

'But I don't have any more time in which to study'; 'I'm already doing X hours a day; I can't do any more'; 'I feel as if my brain is full and isn't taking in any more'—these statements are commonly used when candidates feel like they are not getting anywhere fast. I once made a similar comment to my piano teacher when I was making particularly slow progress. She said 'You don't need to practise for longer, you need to practise properly.' Proper practising meant stopping each time the next note was difficult to find or to play (evidenced by an additional pause) and focussing on this specific note—not the whole bar, not the whole line. Concentrating on the precise part that is difficult, before moving on, makes the studying or practice you are doing more efficient and effective and makes every moment count.

Applying this wisdom to anaesthesia means that while you just want to pass the whole exam, or finish a practice MCQ paper and mark it to see what your score is, you should *stop*. If your mediocre scores are going to change, you need to change something to make this happen. Stop ambling through these questions (the easiest option that counts as studying). Stop at the difficult bits and examine them more closely. Break them down before fitting them all back together again, checking that you have definitely understood them. Stop in this way at each question where your knowledge is incomplete or inadequate. Revert to a textbook and revise the topic in the question. Read all around the questions asked and put them in context. Clarify any bits you do not understand and then go back, answer the question, and move on to the next one. Repeat this process each time you are unsure of an answer. Stop and correct it before moving on. This is proper studying.

This takes a great deal of discipline but makes the time spent more productive and pays huge dividends. It means that the next time you see a rogue question, instead of mumbling 'I always get these ones wrong' you will be confident that you have covered this work and know how to work out the answer.

Say and cover, write and check

Another way to make your studying more effective is to use a technique known to some as SAC WAC (which stands for 'Say and cover, write and check'). This is a technique used in some primary schools to help children learn how to spell and to remember what they have learned.

This technique ensures that rather than merely copying the words from the book to their page, the children must read the word, cover it up and see if they can remember how to spell it, write it down, and then check to see if they were right. When applied to anaesthesia, it springs to mind how easy it is to read a page or a chapter in a textbook and not be able to remember a word of it. Next time that happens, recognize it and correct it. If you are reading a textbook, ensure you are concentrating. At the end of each page ask yourself 'What have I just read?'. Say it out loud. If you cannot say precisely what you have learned, or if you can only say 'It was something about how a vaporizer works', you need to go back and focus on what was actually written. Instead of saying it out loud, you could jot down a few notes, if making notes helps you. Try not to gloss over the hard bits with 'I'll read that another time'. Do it now. Another time will not make it any easier and you will feel no more inclined to do it at a later date.

Repetition and retention

'I can't remember anything for long', and 'If I start too early, I'll have forgotten it all by the time of the exam' are common cries of distress from candidates. Those statements need not be true if you follow a couple of simple rules.

Imagine you have just learned the Bohr equation for calculating physiological dead space. This cannot now be put into the 'completed' pile or it will be forgotten about. You must learn it, then repeat it. Learn it and repeat it. Then write it out several times as the kettle boils at your next break. Repeat it again the next morning as you brush your teeth and make your toast. See if you can remember it an hour later. If not, revise it and keep revisiting it. Why is it you can remember all the words to any ABBA hit single yet cannot remember the Bohr equation? When you accept it is due to the frequency with which you *revisit* the words, you will understand the difference between revision and vision.

If you begin to work your way through the syllabus six months before the exam, you may be worried you will forget some of it. You may well be correct but with your short, frequent, effective studying, you will have time to go through it twice or three times, and each time it will be more memorable, and so will take less time and require less effort.

Decide what type of learner you are

Individuals learn best in different ways, as mentioned at the start of this chapter. Decide which way works best for you. Some prefer traditional reading of a textbook and making revision notes for revisiting, while others make flashcards to carry around. Some learn better from online resources including RCoA and e-learning revision aids, and other, less visually dependent learners find listening to podcasts effective. This can be done while exercising, relaxing, or in the car (but do be very careful if you are driving), making good use of 'dead' time. Some prefer to use exam practice books but, as mentioned earlier, I do not believe that these alone are sufficient or particularly good when learning new subjects.

Using a mixture of revision aids will help you by covering similar topics but in different formats. Using a variety of tools provides a change to your study routine and helps keep boredom at bay.

Set objectives

Decide what you want to achieve by the end of the week, the end of the day, or the end of a two-hour study period. This need not be a large, formal planning task; just jot down what elements of the curriculum you plan to cover in a period of time. This helps keep you focussed and accountable for your time. Knowing that X, Y, and Z have to be covered before stopping will make you progress through topics rather than wasting time day-dreaming at your desk. However, do not allow a never-ending 'to do' list to develop. If your list is too long, you will never get to the end of it, and this will lead to you becoming demoralized. Make your goals achievable and realistic within the time frame. Once completed, you will feel pleased and positive at accomplishing that which you set out to do. Time to reward yourself.

Avoid distractions

It is not true that listening to music, listening to the radio, or having the television on in the background will help you study. It will not. The more inputs there are to the brain, the less attention can be devoted to each one. Switch the radio off and remove the headphones. Similarly, do not be distracted by other tasks. Do not begin to clean your bicycle with a toothbrush, nor paint the spare bedroom. These can wait.

CHAPTER 5

Sort your surroundings

What surrounds us is what is within us.

T.F. Hodge

(Reproduced from T.F. Hodge, from *Within I Rise: Spiritual Triumph over Death and Conscious Encounters with 'The Divine Presence'*, Copyright 2009, with kind permission from America Star Books)

CONTENTS

There is no doubt we are each affected by our surroundings. While preparing for an exam, everything around you should be optimized to facilitate study. There is no need to be diva-like about your requirements: a few essentials are needed and a number of common-sense approaches should be adopted.

Places for studying

You must establish what kind of environment optimizes your studying. Ideally, you would have a dedicated study which would be spacious, bright, and airy, with a large desk and comfortable chair. Most do not have such luxury, so the minimum requirement is somewhere quiet where you will not be interrupted. This may be at home in a study, the dining room, or locked away in the spare bedroom. You may be happiest in a comfortable chair in the lounge but beware of distractions here. Sometimes it is better to be out of the house altogether. Use the public library or the hospital library, particularly if you have small children and arriving home means you are immediately in charge of family life again. Sometimes variety in where you study is good. Wherever you choose, it should be somewhere quiet, where you will not be disturbed or, more importantly, distracted. That means avoiding your mobile phone or computer, as you will find it almost impossible to resist surfing the internet the first time you reach a difficult area or a boring topic. You will *not* ignore texts and you *will* check to see from whom you have a missed call. Ellie Simmonds, the Olympic swimmer, disabled her Twitter account in the run up to the London 2012 Paralympic games to prevent continual tweeting, checking, updating, and so on. This allowed her to focus entirely on her training. Switch your mobile off and reward yourself at the end of the study period by switching it back on.

Do not waste time day-dreaming and do not listen to music or the radio. I do not believe that 'background' music or any other form of white noise is helpful. Earphones are only for listening to podcasts while you travel. (Do not use specific study time for this.) Any additional sensory input to the brain acts as a distraction and makes the brain divide its attention between the matter in hand and the other source. So please, help yourself by finding somewhere quiet.

It is easy to be disturbed if you study close to the kettle and biscuit tin. At every hurdle, it is too easy to get up and make a drink and delay getting to grips with the learning matter. Similarly, will watching ten minutes of the news on television really make a difference? I think it will. You are just distracting yourself, so move away from the temptation of television.

When you get to your place of study, aim to make every moment count when you are there. Ask not to be disturbed (unless with a cup of tea) and focus on the task list for the session. Keep your eye on the prize and remember if you do it right this time, you will not need to do it again.

Keep your study area tidy. A chaotic desk with notes and books strewn everywhere will not help ease your anxieties, but it is useful to have *aide-mémoires* and motivational phrases visible on the wall in front of your desk. Keep your study plan or list visible, too. It is motivating to cross items off as you complete them and helpful in that you can add others to the bottom as they occur to you.

Clear your mind from clutter, too. Write lists of the thoughts, problems, and 'must do' items that pop into your head mid session. Put the lists to one side and deal with them later.

Handling stress

You need time off, too—time when you are free from studying and the obligation to do so. Time off should be planned and delineated rather than occurring by default on those occasions when you cannot be bothered to study. Schedule pleasant things into your week: the cinema, meeting friends, reading a novel, going for a swim, or whatever you enjoy doing. This will give you an incentive to study when you should and to earn time off without guilt.

Looking after your mind is important. Preparing for exams is a huge stressor and you need to find a way to deal with this. Talking about it helps, especially with others in the same boat. Social interaction with peer groups will provide comfort as you learn you are not the only one suffering. Another mode of learning is to arrange to study together, at times. By asking each other questions, you can practise for SOEs and learn from hearing the way someone else presents a topic. You can even ask them questions on topics about which you are not confident and learn the answers, too!

Hopefully, partners will be sympathetic to your doom and gloom (although this will not last indefinitely). Speak to your colleagues and consultants. You will not be the first stressed out exam candidate the department has seen (nor will you be the last) and they will understand the pressure. Departmental secretaries are always good for a cup of tea and a biscuit if you are lucky. They usually have tissues too, when it all becomes too much.

If it really is becoming too much, you may need to take a step back and consider your health. You can discuss your health and well-being, in confidence, with your general practitioner or the occupational health service in your hospital. If you need more pastoral care, you can approach your college tutor or someone else whom you trust with your woes.

Staying healthy

Aim to preserve your health and well-being where possible. Tempting though it may be to reward yourself with a glass of wine or a bottle of beer at the end of every evening, you will pay the price the next day and the next, and as the days and weeks pass, residual alcohol will accumulate and make you feel awful. Feeling any less than 100% will only make your task harder and will zap your energy and motivation. Try to avoid alcohol in the run-up to the exam. It will still be there, chilled and waiting for you afterwards.

Try to eat well. Whether you believe we are what we eat, or we get out what we put in, do not choose to eat junk. There are plenty of fast-food options that are not junk food if you have a microwave. Try and stick to your usual meal times too. Missing meals and snacking on crisps and chocolate to 'save time' will not help you in the long run. You know all about stable blood glucose levels versus excess sugar spikes, insulin splurges, and resounding crashes. It is basic but try and be kind to your body to help it work well for you. Give it wholesome, balanced nutrition.

Adequate sleep

Similarly with caffeine, do not be tempted to take caffeine tablets to keep you alert or awake for longer in an attempt to help you study. It, too, peaks and crashes leaving you feeling worse. Remember, this is a marathon not a sprint and whatever way you study needs to be sustainable. By planning ahead and beginning early enough, you can get through the work without resorting to nocturnal hours.

If you usually drink a lot of coffee or soft drinks containing caffeine, it may affect your sleep and you may want to consider limiting these or avoiding them later in the day. You will have plenty of endogenous catecholamines to keep you alert and focussed.

Even if it is difficult to sleep well, ensure you allow enough time for sleep. Numerous studies show we learn better if we are well rested. Staying up later and later to study does not pay dividends in the long term. The advice for getting to sleep when your brain is buzzing with facts, ideas, and questions is to allow it time to calm down beforehand. Schedule some time to unwind between finishing studying and going to bed. Relax as you wish. Having a long bath works for some. If you can go swimming after studying, this is a great stress reliever and relaxant. It also leaves you feeling physically tired as well as mentally exhausted and helps you sleep better.

Take some leave

If possible, book some leave in the weeks prior to the exam. Private study leave will be at the discretion of your department but there is no harm in asking. Annual leave ought to be granted if booked far enough in advance and will give you time to study or visit different clinical areas and gives the added assurance that you will not be doing a week of night shifts immediately before the exam.

If you have leave to spare, request a few days off afterwards if you feel you need time to relax or pay attention to other areas in your life. Having a holiday to look forward to can be a great incentive. Imagine going away somewhere exotic knowing that you have passed your exam and that it is not just a quick pit stop until you return home and begin studying all over again.

Exercise

Exercise is beneficial, as we all know, but it is also a good way to relieve stress and frustration and deal with excess circulating adrenaline. Try to find an exercise you enjoy (if such a thing exists) and if you hate the gym, do not go! Swimming is good, or going for a run or a brisk walk can be enjoyable and just as effective. It is particularly cathartic when it is raining. Try it. You will not dissolve.

Mind management

Be disciplined and follow your timetable for study and relaxation time. Knowing you are well prepared will reduce your fear and anxiety and leave room for you to develop a positive attitude. This is your exam—and it is your exam to pass. No one will fail you, but you may fail yourself. You need to develop self-belief. You need to get psyched! Get mad even! You have paid a lot of money and spent a lot of time studying and preparing, now is your pay-back time. It is your turn to show the examiners all that you know. Do not be afraid. Be happy that the day has arrived and do not hold back.

On the day

Pay attention to the basic logistics and avoid schoolboy errors. Where is the exam? Which building? How are you going to travel there? What will you do if there are roadworks and traffic jams or leaves on the line and frozen points? You need a plan B.

Plan A may be to stay somewhere close by, the night before the exam. If you do so, go out the evening before the exam and get your bearings. (Hotels in London often have more than one exit onto different streets, so please be sure to know the direction in which to go.) Get as good a night's sleep as possible but if you cannot sleep in a strange bed in a noisy city, do not worry. A little adrenaline improves performance, so pre-exam nerves are actually helping you. Obviously, get up early and leave far more time than usual for breakfast and plenty of time for checking out of the hotel. You can leave any luggage at the hotel or alternatively store it in a locker at the RCoA.

I advise against last-minute revision. I cannot think of any benefit to desperately flicking through a handbook or a stack of revision notes while waiting to enter the exam hall. Do not worry if you cannot remember a specific fact. Your time is better spent calming yourself down. Take deep breaths and concentrate on breathing out. Strike up a conversation with the person next to you (they will be feeling as anxious as you are) and talk about anything except anaesthesia to pass the time. Make sure you are wearing a watch and obey the current rules concerning what items you can and cannot take into the exam with you.

There is no need to wish you good luck. You have studied hard and created your own luck. Remember you can only do your best.

PART 2

THE PRIMARY FRCA

CHAPTER 6

The Multiple Choice Question (MCQ) and Single Best Answer (SBA) paper

CONTENTS

The Primary FRCA examination is blue printed to the Basic Level Training Curriculum (http://rcoa.ac.uk/node/207). In Annex B of the 2010 Curriculum, the core learning outcomes are listed for each unit of training. These consist of knowledge, skills, and attitudes to be achieved. They are listed along with a column denoting how each competency can be assessed. Those knowledge competences suffixed by the letter 'E' are assessed via examination and together form the syllabus for the Primary exam. Questions from a unit of training may appear in any component of the exam. Table 6.1 shows an example of some knowledge competencies as listed in Annex B.

All questions in FRCA exams are mapped to the relevant competencies within the curriculum. This means that, when selecting questions for exam papers, the examiners are able to ensure a broad sampling of the entire curriculum and that each sitting of the exam is balanced to ensure that all areas are covered.

The Primary exam consists of a stand alone written paper comprising multiple choice questions (MCQs) and single best answer questions (SBAs). This is followed by the Objective Structured Clinical Exam (OSCE) and the Structured Oral Exams (SOEs). In this chapter, we discuss the MCQ/SBA paper. In addition, please read Chapter 8, as you will find more advice there which is relevant to both the Primary and the Final MCQ/SBA papers.

Requirements of the MCQ/SBA paper

This paper lasts three hours and usually takes place in the afternoon at several regional centres throughout the UK. There are currently three sittings of this exam each year. A maximum of six attempts are permitted and a pass is valid for three years. Further details are available on the website (http://www.rcoa.ac.uk/examinations).

The paper consists of 60 true/false (T/F) MCQs and 30 SBA questions. There is no requirement to pass each component individually, so a poor score in one area can be compensated for by a better performance in another. Questions are devised to sample all parts of the 2010 Curriculum for Basic Training in Anaesthesia.

Table 6.1 Knowledge competencies listed for day surgery in basic anaesthesia

Knowledge competence	Description	Assessment methods
DS_BK_08	Describes appropriate analgesia for day cases.	A, C, E
DS_BK_09	Describes strategies to reduce post-operative nausea and vomiting in day-case patients.	A, C, E
DS_BK_10	Explains the management and assessment of recovery of day-surgery patients to street fitness.	A, C, E

The MCQs have one stem and five leaves, A to E, which require an answer of true or false. There is no negative marking: a correct answer receives a score of +1 and an incorrect answer receives a score of 0. There is no value in missing out any questions and all 300 should be answered.

The pass rate for this paper hovers at around 70%. The exam is a test of knowledge and the significant failure rate reflects a lack of knowledge in one or more areas of the curriculum. There is a lot you must learn if you are to pass and no escaping the fact that a significant amount of studying is required. It is useful to think about how you learn best. Some prefer to read books, while others can learn from a computer screen, a smartphone app, or by listening to a pod cast. Individuals have different preferences. Some make notes, some highlight their textbooks, and others prefer to simply read. It is best to use a combination of techniques. A multi-modal approach means you can chop and change between different ways of studying and prevent boredom, and allows for the fact that different topics can be better taught and learned one way rather than another. The rest of this chapter will look at some different ways of studying for the MCQ paper.

A common complaint from candidates is that much of what they are required to know is not clinically relevant. The way to make these facts memorable is to identify *how* they *are* relevant and 'hang' these facts onto patients or events occurring in theatre.

The tools of our trade are drugs, equipment, and the human body. It is vital we have an understanding of how each works and interacts with the others if we are to anaesthetize patients safely and successfully. Plumbers know how flow through tubes can change; chefs and scientists know what happens when different compounds are mixed together. Anaesthetists, however, must factor in a huge variable—the action and reaction of the human body in maintaining homeostasis while managing insults and stress. Knowledge of normal function in health is vital. Knowing the effects that drugs have on the body (pharmacodynamics) must be known in order to adapt our use of them in patients with ill health. We *must* understand *how* our equipment works and how it may fail. It is as important to know the limitations and errors associated with our equipment as to know the way it can monitor our patients accurately and support their breathing by replicating physiological respiration.

Pharmacology is often reported as being especially difficult by Primary exam candidates. This is largely due to their underestimating the *depth* of knowledge that is required. It is difficult to learn factual values for an endless number of drugs when the relevance of these to clinical practice is questioned, but these values *are* clinically relevant. They reveal why the action of different drugs is variable in differing patient populations. I agree it is hard to learn and remember lots of numbers and values, and I will provide some suggestions as to how this task may be made easier.

It is reasonable to expect candidates to have an extensive, in-depth knowledge of all drugs that they administer to patients each day, including finer points of detail. Knowing that propofol comes as a 20 ml glass vial containing a white emulsified solution of 10 mg/ml to be given at a dose of 2–3 mg/kg is not enough. Candidates must be aware of its physicochemical, pharmacodynamic, and pharmacokinetic properties, as well as its interactions and unwanted effects in order to anticipate the actions and manage the reactions occurring in their patients.

Make lists

When learning a series of values, you should round the numbers to ballpark figures and remember these. Note the value at the mid-point of the scale and the relative values of other drugs above and below this number. In MCQs that ask if particular values are true or false, you will know if they are *around* the correct level. For example, you may be asked if the following are true/false about drug X:

a. 17% is excreted unchanged in the urine
b. Has a bioavailability of 92%
c. 45% is protein-bound
d. Is more potent than drug Y
e. Has low potential for histamine release

While you may not know these *absolute* values, you should have a working knowledge of whether the drugs you administer are highly protein-bound, have a high bioavailability, or commonly cause histamine release.

I suggest you learn some extreme examples by making lists. Get a little notebook to carry around with you and make lists of drugs under various headings of your choosing, but including features such as:

● High protein binding
● Low protein binding
● Contraindicated in porphyria
● Triggers for malignant hyperpyrexia
● Interaction with warfarin
● Induces hepatic enzymes
● Potentiates the action of non-depolarizing muscle relaxants

Arrange them alphabetically or create a pneumonic that you will remember—it does not have to make sense; it only needs to be memorable to you. Identify drugs that appear in more than one list and look for features that are common to more than one drug.

Making lists per se will not help you to learn the facts. You must use them. You must *look at them* frequently. Read them; cover them; say them; and repeat them. Challenge yourself to remember all the contents of a list. Use them in theatre in this way when you are alone or give them to your consultant to test you when you have an accompanied list. Promise incentives to yourself. Simple rewards, such as a cake at lunchtime if you recall all lists correctly, will make you smile and, crucially, keep your motivation high to learn some more.

Make tables

You can also learn and remember facts, relative to each other, by ranking them in your mind. Tables often help and you can easily make these (see Tables 6.2 and 6.3) and carry them in your pocket or purse. This is rote learning with the addition of *aide-mémoirs*. You should look at the tables each time you have two minutes to spare. Challenge yourself!

You can order the top row of drugs to see a pattern to the numbers and properties of each agent running from left to right or right to left. You need not remember every single value but if you look at it often enough, you will remember where different values lie and how they relate to those around them in the table. You will know approximations of some values and you will be able to deduce many more. Some will stick in your memory for different reasons: values close to those in neighbouring boxes, others having vastly different values despite being in the same class,

Table 6.2 Physical and pharmacological properties of volatile anaesthetic agents

	Halothane	Isoflurane	Enflurane	Sevoflurane	Desflurane
MAC	0.75	1.15	1.68	2–3	6–10
M. wt	197	184.5	184.5	200	168
BP	50.2	48.5	56.5	58.5	23.5
B/G	2.5	1.4	1.91	0.6	0.42
O/W coeff.	220	174	120	53	18.7
SVP@20	32kPa	32kPa	23.3kPa	21.3kPa	88.5
Metabolism	20% liver	0.2% liver	2.4%	3% cyt P450	0.02%
Specific features	Sensitizes heart to A,NA; hepatitis risk with repeated use	Suitable for epileptics; potentiates NDMR +	Fluoride conc. high; avoid in epileptics	Potentiates NDMR + +	Paradoxical tachycardia if dose rapidly increased

and others just stick for no specific reason. Look out for your door number or year of birth appearing in this context. This method will help you remember many facts and figures required in the MCQ paper. The key is to revisit your tables frequently. This is an easy thing to do in a short period of otherwise 'dead' time.

Identify your reference drug to give you a meaningful benchmark onto which you can hang the subsequent values. For example, Table 6.2 shows the volatile agents. I use isoflurane as my reference; it was the first volatile agent I used regularly, and I still think in terms of its equivalence, but you can choose whichever drug you prefer. You can then relate the pharmacological values of other agents to their clinical effects which you already know, and in relation to your reference drug. From Table 6.2, note the decreasing blood–gas partition coefficient from left to right. This

Table 6.3 Pharmacological properties of opioids

	Morphine	Diamorphine	Alfentanil	Remifentanil	Fentanyl
Relative potency	1	1.8	1	150–200	100
Duration of action	3–4 hours; peak at 5–10 mins	3–4 hours	5–10 mins; peak at 90 secs	3–10 mins	40–300 mins
Elimination half life (mins)	90–240	2–3	100	10–30	30
Protein binding (%)	20–40	No	85–92	70	81–94
Metabolism	M3G,M6G (active)	To morphine initially	N-dealkylation	Hydrolysis by esterases	N-dealkylation
Pro-drug?	No	Yes	No	No	No
Specific features				TCI context sensitive t1/2	Duration of action varies with dose

corresponds to speed of onset and offset, which you know from experience. Note that the boiling point of desflurane is anomalous: this is why it requires a different type of vapourizer, which you know. (Can you explain how it works?) All the others have boiling-point values in the same ballpark. So, in the MCQ 'concerning isoflurane', asking if the boiling point is 48.9, you know they are all around 50 and the answer is therefore true.

Look for similarities, too. Sevoflurane and halothane have similar molecular weights. Isoflurane and enflurane are isomers and, therefore, have the same molecular weight and their saturated vapour pressures (SVPs) have the same numbers, only in reverse order. Notable points like this make otherwise meaningless values memorable.

By doing this type of pattern and analysis, you will be able to deduce many answers and make highly educated guesses for questions to which you are unsure of the correct answer.

'Specific features' (see last row of Table 6.2) give you something additional that you know about to bring up in an SOE.

In the equivalent table for opioids, morphine is the standard drug which can be used as a comparator for all other opioids (see Table 6.3).

Clear your mind

Many question stems are of the format: Compared to drug X, drug Y has a *greater or lesser*:

a. Elimination half life

b. Speed of onset

c. Side-effect profile

d. Histamine-releasing potential

e. Degree of metabolism

It is important to read these questions accurately and slowly and be clear in your mind what is being asked *before* you begin to answer any of them. To prevent confusion (or confusing yourself!), stop reading the question where it states 'drug Y'. Cover the five leaves below, and jot down all the values you can remember for both drugs X and Y, or actually write out which is more potent than the other, etc. Now you have the facts securely written down and these are not subject to the gymnastics going on in your mind about whether a higher pKa will cause more or less protein binding or if a greater pH means it is more or less acidic.

These questions are not deliberately convoluted, nor are they intended to be a test of English comprehension. They can be confusing though, and they can be easily changed. Those which you remember from practice papers may not be exactly the same questions and the answers will certainly not be the same. I cannot stress enough that you must read the questions carefully and do not allow yourself to 'recognize it and skip quickly' onto the answers.

I prepared tables for local anaesthetic drugs (see Table 6.4) and general anaesthetic induction agents. If I was sitting the exam now, I would prepare a table for new anticoagulant and antiplatelet drugs, detailing their half lives, metabolism, actions, and reversal strategies.

There will, no doubt, be similar tables available online and many candidates may consider pieces of handwritten paper unnecessary (even if highlighted and laminated!) because they have the tables 'saved on their phone'. This may be true but, personally, I find it easier to remember what I am learning if I have constructed the table and looked up the values myself. I find a paper copy easier to justify looking at in the anaesthetic room or in theatre. It makes a bad impression if you are seen to be fiddling constantly with your phone. Finally, as mentioned in Chapter 3, electronic devices provide many distractions and are to be discouraged when the focus is on exam preparation.

Table **6.4** Pharmacological properties of local anaesthetics

	Lignocaine	Bupivicaine	Ropivicaine	Cocaine
Max dose mg/kg	3	0.5	3	3
pKa	7.1	8.2	8.1	8.6
Protein binding	64%	95%	94%	98%
Elimination half life (mins)	100	30–60	60–180	60
Amide/ester	Amide	Amide	Amide	Ester

Repetition

As well as learning the lists you have made, you should read about the drugs you use, each and every time you use them. This way you read about commonly used drugs more frequently than you do about rarely used drugs, and will learn and remember more facts about drugs you use most frequently and you will know, at least something about those drugs you use less frequently.

The best way to do this is with a pocket-sized pharmacology book. *Drugs in anaesthesia and intensive care* by M. Sasada and S. Smith is commonly used for this purpose as, for each drug, it provides a two-page spread covering the physicochemical, pharmacodynamic, and pharmacokinetic properties and values. Following the same systematic approach to each drug provides you with mental 'prompts' to help recall information. It also provides a framework on which to hang an answer in the SOEs, and you should bear this format in mind. Read the pages, close the book, and try to verbalize what you have just read.

Use this book *between* patients to make use of this dead time, particularly out of hours. As you wait for the patient to be brought to the anaesthetic room, read the relevant pages for the drugs you have prepared for use. This makes perfect revision sense and good use of otherwise wasted time on call.

Depending on the edition of the book, there may or may not be certain newer drugs included, so do not rely solely on this as a comprehensive guide to peri-operative pharmacology. If you do not have this book, then buy or borrow it while you are studying. If you forget to bring it with you, read the patient information leaflets found inside the boxes. These contain a surprising amount of information which is more relevant to you than the patient.

Start with the general anaesthesia drugs and progress to analgesics, antiemetics, antibiotics, antithrombotics, insulin, steroids, and any other drug you may give in theatre. When the patient is stable, look up all the drugs on their prescription chart. What are they each for? What are their interactions? What are their side-effects, their pharmacodynamics, their special points?

Study smarter

Do not waste time trying to question-spot. Instead, take a general overview. Common things occur commonly, and commonly used drugs crop up in exams. It is easy to identify topics most likely to be included. What would you ask if you were setting the paper? What topics would you least like to answer? Identify these and rectify this!

Tricyclic antidepressants (TCAs), selective serotonin re-uptake inhibitors (SSRIs), and monoamine oxidase inhibitors (MAOIs) are often asked about, particularly with regard to concomitant use of different vasopressors, epinephrine, and antimuscarinics.

The prevalence of diabetes is rising in the UK, so knowledge about insulin (infusions and glucose, potassium, and insulin (GKI) regimes) and traditional, as well as newer, oral hypoglycaemic agents should be covered. The obesity epidemic continues and with it the risk of peri-operative deep vein thrombosis or pulmonary thromboembolism. Anticoagulants—from heparin and warfarin, through low molecular weight heparins, to newer oral anticoagulants—are likely topics to be included in the MCQ.

Cardiovascular and cerebrovascular events are prevented using antiplatelet drugs and many patients present on aspirin, and dipyridamole. These, and newer agents such as ticagrelor, are all fair questions in this exam. Suggammadex and muscle relaxants will be asked about. Think about how to use them and when they cannot be used. What if the patient has to return to theatre from recovery?

Questions about basic sciences are absolutely right or wrong, true or false, so to test application of knowledge in a clinical context, a scenario may be used. This is also the case in the SBA section of this paper.

Practising MCQs

Practising MCQs from books and websites forms a large part of many candidates' preparation. This is good: if you are going to race hurdles, you should train for hurdles after all. However, such practice must be used properly to gain maximal benefit from your time and effort. It is very easy to 'have a go' at a few questions, check the answers, spot your mistakes, and move on. Indeed, many candidates do this as an easier option when they are not in the mood for studying proper. If you wait until you are in the right mood for studying before doing any, you may wait a long time. Focus your mind into studying mode and remember that this is like anything else where what you get out is only as good as what you put in.

When you do practise MCQ papers, I suggest you do them in batches of ten (stems). Practise reading them accurately and write your answers down. As you mark them and find an incorrect answer, do not merely accept that you got it wrong and then try to remember the correct response. This will not work when doing so many questions and it will not work when a similar, but slightly different, question comes up in the future, as you will be considering what you *thought* was the correct answer and what actually *was* the correct answer and, ultimately, will be guessing yet again.

What you should do is go back to the basics of the topic in question. For example, consider the question: Gas flow through a tube is affected by:

a. Temperature
b. Viscosity
c. Molecular weight
d. Length of tube
e. Diameter of tube

If you do not answer all five correctly, do not simply make a list, from these options, of the variables affecting flow. The list is not exhaustive and the question may reappear with five different options. Instead, go back to a physics and measurement textbook and revise flow through tubes. Learn gas flow, liquid flow, viscosity, density, features of different tubes in anaesthesia, flow meters, flow at altitude, and so on. Read the whole subject and put the individual facts into context of the complete topic. This way, when you see this question (or a similar one) again, you will either know the answer or have a better knowledge base on which to begin working it out.

This is time-consuming and requires self-discipline to do. It is very tempting to speed through a whole MCQ paper and mark it quickly (but then bemoan your score). Now you have identified gaps in your knowledge you should remedy them as best you possibly can. This is not by memorizing random facts from the answer section of MCQ books.

The SBA section

The SBAs are a different type of assessment than MCQs. Instead of testing only the narrow 'knows' element of knowledge, the SBAs test the wider 'knows how' and 'knows why' elements. They have an increased ability to discriminate between pass and fail candidates as a higher range of marks are available. They were introduced to the FRCA in September 2011 when, on the advice of the Postgraduate Medical Education and Training Board (PMETB), the RCoA agreed to modernize the exam and to bring it into line with most other medical exam boards. The introduction of SBAs was seen as a chance to improve the exam.

Basic science, as tested in the Primary FRCA, is factual knowledge. It is definitely either true or false, and thus often does not lend itself well to an SBA question. This has led to many basic science questions in the Primary FRCA being framed within a given clinical scenario. This should make it easier for candidates as it then becomes directly relevant to clinical practice.

In the SBA questions, you must choose one option from A to E which is the *best* answer to the question. Please note that this is NOT an A to E multiple choice where there is *only* one correct answer. In SBA questions, there may appear to be several acceptable answers within the A to E options; some may be plausible and several may be possible. However, there will be one answer that is *better* than the others, most usually for objective reasons which are referenced to evidence or guidelines in sources familiar to candidates at this level of experience.

When you pass this paper, you have up to three years in which to sit the OSCE and SOEs. Do not delay this unnecessarily.

CHAPTER 7

The Objective Structured Clinical Exam (OSCE) and Structured Oral Exams (SOEs)

The OSCE and SOE must be taken together at the first attempt. When one of the two is passed, then only the outstanding part needs to be taken at the next sitting. Where both are failed, they must be retaken together.

The OSCE

Just as viva practice is the best way to prepare for a SOE, a practice OSCE is an invaluable means of revising for the OSCE. Many schools have developed and run a practice OSCE for candidates but, if not, aim to attend one elsewhere, using your study leave and budget.

The OSCE is the only part of the exam where your application of knowledge can be tested and it is very much a clinical exam. There are 17 stations, lasting 1 hour 42 minutes; 5 minutes per station is usual. At the time of writing, stations include resuscitation, technical skills, anatomy, history taking, physical examination, communication skills, anaesthetic hazards, and the interpretation of X-rays. There is usually a simulation station utilizing a medium-fidelity simulator.

The OSCE is continually evolving as new stations are developed to reflect up-to-date ways of working and new ways of learning. Many stations are unmanned and, in some, you will give your answers using a touch screen to answer 'True' or 'False'. All stations have instructions to read, located outside the booths, before the exam period begins. These are very clear and explicit. You should stay calm and read them accurately. Be sure to understand what the question is specifically asking. Others will have X-rays or computed tomography (CT) scans which are displayed on screen (as opposed to light boxes), reflecting the change to online radiology. Anatomy stations may utilize part task trainers, photographs, or pictures of the area in question. Surface anatomy may be tested on a live model.

There will be a resuscitation station. Be sure to confirm which version of the Resuscitation Council UK Guidelines are being used for your exam. You must know the algorithms for adults and children and be proficient in basic and advanced life support, as you will be asked to demonstrate one of these. For this station, your attire must be sensible and comfortable. Do not begin the OSCE circuit trussed up in a three-piece suit or wearing your highest heels and tightest skirt. There are no marks for sartorial elegance but there may well be marks for procedures which require you to kneel down beside the mannikin, pull him into the recovery position, or perform chest compressions. If you are wearing a suit, remove your jacket at the beginning. This is a time when comfort must prevail over fashion.

There will be station(s) with actors, to assess history taking and communication skills. It should hardly need to be stated that you must be professional and correct at these stations. Always begin by introducing yourself to the patient and checking that you have the correct patient. (Don't forget hand hygiene.) Remember they may be terrified, worried, aggressive, or complaining and you should manage each of these scenarios. Be honest if the patient asks you something you do not know, but reassure them you will ask someone who can answer their question. Give the patient opportunity to ask you their questions and, if they are reticent, sometimes managing their silence with silence allows them to air their concerns. Ask for permission from the patient before any examination, including that of the airway, and if you are going to touch the patient, ask to wash your hands before and after, or to use alcohol gel.

You will have completed your intensive care unit of training in advance of this exam, so make sure you have had plenty of practice at interpreting arterial blood gases and pressure volume loops. This is true for electrocardiograms (ECGs), also. Make sure you practice reporting ECGs in a formal driving-test style. For example: 'This is a 12-lead ECG of Mr A. The paper speed is B and the quality is C'. Ignore any diagnosis made by the machine; it may be wrong. Next, systematically comment upon the axis, rate, rhythm (sinus or non-sinus at first). Progress to the P waves, the QRS complex, ST segments and T waves, stating whether these are normal or not in terms of length and morphology. Lastly, comment upon any outstanding features that you spot. This is often the diagnosis but you must not rush straight to it or you will risk missing out important accessory information. An ECG will most likely be an unmanned station with a question paper for you to answer. Habitually reporting ECGs using this framework means you will be thorough and confident of your findings.

The SOE

SOE 1

In the Primary FRCA, the SOE consists of two subsections. The first 30 minutes comprises three questions in pharmacology and three questions in physiology and biochemistry. As with the multiple-choice element, do not underestimate the depth of knowledge required, particularly in pharmacology. You will be asked about drugs you administer commonly and those with significant or important interactions. In my opinion, monoamine oxidase inhibitors are one of the favourites. Newer drugs also appear in exams. Currently, suggammadex is still topical, and we now see patients treated with newer oral antidiabetic and anticoagulant drugs by general practitioners (GPs) which have important ramifications in the peri-operative period. You may be asked to talk about a drug you use regularly in clinical practice. This is a golden opportunity. Choose which drugs you will talk about in advance. Prepare one from each of several categories, prior to the exam, and know everything about them. You should present this knowledge systematically, under these headings:

- Physical and chemical properties
- Indications, dose, and administration
- Pharmacodynamic features (what the drug does to the body)
  - Cardiovascular
  - Respiratory
  - Gastrointestinal
  - Genitourinary
  - Central nervous system
  - Haemopoetic system

- Pharmacokinetic information (what the body does to the drug)
  - Absorption
  - Distribution
  - Metabolism
  - Excretion
- Special points to note

By this point, the examiners will be impressed and possibly bored by your organized recital of pharmacology. It takes only a little preparation and practice beforehand to allow you to pass with confidence.

When using the systems approach for pharmacodynamics, be sure to include *all* systems affected. Many candidates stop after the cardiovascular and respiratory systems, forgetting to mention the effects on the central nervous system, the gut, the genitourinary system, and blood dyscrasias which may occur. Pharmacokinetics are described under the four headings as listed and you should know at least some of the numerical values.

There are a few definitions you should know verbatim for the SOE:

- Half life of a drug
- Clearance
- Volume of distribution
- The Munro-Kelly doctrine
- The pKa
- The Fick principle

These easily become muddled under stress.

Equations which you should practise writing out repeatedly beforehand include:

- Hagen-Poiseuille equation
- Shunt equation
- Bernoulli's equation
- Nernst equation
- Henderson-Hasselbach equation
- The alveolar–arterial (A–a) gradient and alveolar gas equation

In addition, there are several graphs you should be able to produce voluntarily and accurately which will show your answers perhaps better than you can explain them. You must label both axes, showing the units of measurement. It is polite to ask if you may draw a diagram. Examples include:

- Concentration–time graph for various drugs and routes of administration
- Three graphs relating intracranial pressure (ICP) with intracranial volume (ICV), pO2, and pCO2 and mean arterial pressure (MAP)
- A normal capnography tracing with inflections labelled
- Waveforms of the cardiac cycle and the jugular venous pressure (JVP)
- Heart rate (HR) and MAP variation during a valsalva manoeuvre

These lists are by no means exhaustive and you should add to them as you progress through Annex B of the basic training curriculum.

SOE 2

In the second 30 minutes, there are three questions on physics, clinical measurement, equipment and safety, and three questions on clinical topics, one of which will include a critical incident. The clinical topic will be of a standard relevant to a trainee completing basic training. Any critical incident at this level demands that senior help be called, regardless of other commitments they may be purported to have. You must state this explicitly in the exam, remembering it is better to call for help sooner rather than later.

Preparing for the SOE

The SOE is the most feared part of any exam. Indeed, part of the test is managing your anxiety in a stressful situation. To be able to compute a clear and sensible answer, despite feeling terrified and unsure, is a sign of clinical competency.

The first thing you must achieve is control of your mind. You should not become timid, afraid, shut down, and terrified that you do not know anything. Give yourself credit for the hours of study and preparation you have put into this exam and reassure yourself that you can do your best. Be aware of your heightened adrenaline levels and harness them to increase your determination and improve your performance. The best way to deal with an incredibly stressful situation is to make a plan for dealing with it in advance—a plan that you have practised so many times, it is ingrained in your memory to the extent it can happen automatically.

Think of performing a rapid sequence induction. The moment you realize you cannot visualize the larynx, your stress level increases exponentially. This is not the time to be considering your options. Your options and actions are pre-defined, pre-agreed, pre-planned. You will attempt intubation once or twice more while correcting head/pillow position and optimizing assistance and equipment. After that, you will declare a failed intubation and call for help. Next, you will oxygenate the patient either via a facemask or a laryngeal mask airway until they awaken. You learned this in advance of working without direct supervision so that when it happens, you can activate and follow this drill and manage the situation without having to make complicated decisions in your moment of stress.

In terms of the SOE, this comes back to having real-time practice with the most intimidating colleagues you can find, as often as possible. It is far better to make your mistakes and become tongue-tied in advance, when it does not count as an attempt at the exam. The more you practise, the less anxious you will feel at the beginning of each session. Candidates who do this report feeling relaxed in the actual exam; they find the examiners to be welcoming and pleasant and much less intimidating (despite being unknown to them).The same principle applies to preparing for an interview for specialty training (and for your consultant post). You must practise exactly what you are required to produce on the day. It never gets any easier but practice does indeed make perfect.

You must be proactive about arranging viva practice and get over your fear of looking stupid and feeling embarrassed in front of senior colleagues. They have all been there, too, and will be aware of your pain. Even well-prepared candidates find practice vivas an ordeal. Practice vivas are a vital part of preparation for the SOE and the sooner you begin to do this, the better prepared you will be. Familiarity reduces anxiety and practising in as close a situation as possible to the actual exam is the best way to sound fluent and confident and to learn to think on your feet.

College tutors, educational supervisors, and other consultants are all busy and many do not know when exams take place. Do not wait for your trainers to suggest viva practice. Better to approach individuals in advance. The reason for this, particularly for the Primary FRCA exam, is that many consultants have forgotten the level of knowledge required about processes not used in daily clinical practice and, therefore, appreciate having time to do some preparation. Seek practice from as many different anaesthetists as possible. This way you will see a variety of examiner styles as well as visit and revisit a diverse range of topics from the syllabus (since each consultant has their own favourite questions to ask).

You may find that the 'examiners' are stern, unfriendly, and apparently unimpressed by your answers. They may be writing things down and appearing not to listen. Alternatively, they may be warm and friendly, helpful even, nodding as you answer, and prompting you if you need help. Do not infer anything from either of these personas. They may be deliberate or unintentional, but do not be guided by them. Do not expect the examiner to endorse your answer or positively reinforce it. Similarly, think carefully if asked 'Are you sure?'. You should take this question at face value. It does not necessarily mean you have got it wrong or that the examiners are trying to trick you. It does show, however, if you have made a lucky guess that turned out to be correct.

Through practice, you will find gaps in your knowledge and areas where your knowledge is not of sufficient depth or detail. This is good, so do not be disheartened. Once identified, these deficiencies can be corrected. When you find such gaps, remedy them at the first opportunity. Do not allow them to accumulate on a list 'to be learned before exam'. When I prepare candidates for the exam, having found a topic they do not know, I take note of it. The next time we meet up, I start with that same question. Often, it has not yet been covered and, when that is the case, I know it will be very difficult to help motivate that person when they cannot motivate themselves.

It is your viva, so you should be doing most of the talking, while keeping the ball in play. It is also your viva to do with as you wish. It is yours to pass or fail. The examiners will not fail you. Only you can cause yourself to fail, so stay calm, pause before you answer the question, and do not panic. Start with the basics and see where the follow-up questions direct you. You have studied hard and paid (a lot of) money to take this exam. This is your opportunity to show the examiners how much you know and how well you know it, and then to invite them to ask you another question and test you on another area of the curriculum.

It is a bit like a tennis match, where the ball is being hit back and forth over the net. When the examiners serve it into your court, you must deal with it correctly and efficiently, and send it back to them without further ado. Make them ask you another question. Remind yourself not to keep talking on and on while your voice fades away in an increasingly unsure tone. Do not give your answer as a question to the examiner, for example 'Is it because . . . ?'. This shows you are unsure and will detract from a correct answer while flagging an area of weakness in your knowledge which the examiners may decide to explore in more detail. Speaking quietly or slowly does not make the words you are saying any more likely to be correct. So give your answer confidently, then stop talking. The examiners will let you know if they would like more detail on what you have said or if they wish to change the topic. Talking indefinitely increases the chance of wandering into dangerous territory where you are unsure of facts.

You must tread a fine line when answering, between responding extensively in all directions and having to have the answer dragged from you with continual prompting from the examiners. Say too much and you risk being asked more about a topic you mentioned transiently, yet of which you have no concrete knowledge. The converse is that continual prompting for each answer will reduce your score from a pass (+ 2 marks) to borderline (+ 1 mark). The way to find this balance is, yet again, through practice, during which you will learn to 'read' the examiners. As you begin to answer the question in a broad sense, you may be encouraged to continue, directed towards one of the categories you have mentioned, or you may be asked a more direct question, to obtain the correct answer. Practise what you will say when you do not know the answer. 'I'm sorry, can you repeat the question?' or 'I'm sorry, my mind has gone blank. Can we come back to that question?' are acceptable requests when stress is preventing you from thinking clearly.

There are video recordings available on the RCoA website showing a candidate perform in the SOE. There are examples of a 'pass' performance and of a 'borderline' performance. Both make very informative viewing. You should study these in addition to all the other resources for candidates on the website.

After the OSCE and SOE

When you pass the OSCE and SOE, you will have passed the full Primary FRCA and will be eligible to apply for ST posts. You should plan ahead to the Final FRCA exams and consider when may be the best time for you to attempt these. The full Primary remains valid for seven years but most candidates take the Final FRCA exams within the following three years.

THE FINAL FRCA

The MCQ/SBAs paper

CONTENTS

The Final FRCA exam is blue printed to the Intermediate Level Training Curriculum (http://rcoa. ac.uk/node/208). In Annex C of the 2010 Curriculum, the core learning outcomes are listed for each unit of training. These consist of knowledge, skills, and attitudes to be achieved. They are listed in a series of tables, along with a column denoting how each competence can be assessed. Knowledge competencies have the letter 'E' in the assessment column which shows they are assessed by exam. They can be tested in any aspect of the exam. Therefore, the curriculum's knowledge competencies marked by the letter 'E' make up the exam syllabus. Table 8.1 shows an example of competences listed in Annex C.

All questions used in FRCA exams are mapped to the relevant competencies within the curriculum. This means that when selecting questions for exam papers, the examiners are able to guarantee a broad sampling of the entire curriculum and that each sitting of the exam will be balanced to ensure all areas are covered. Questions from a unit of training may appear in any component of the exam.

The written paper for the Final FRCA consists of a Short Answer Question (SAQ) paper in the morning and the MCQ/SBA paper in the afternoon. If you are preparing for the Final FRCA, make sure you go back and reread Chapter 6, where you will find additional advice that is relevant to both the Primary and the Final MCQ/SBA papers.

To pass the written part of the FRCA you must achieve the pass mark for the SAQ and the MCQ/SBA papers combined. Therefore, doing particularly well in one paper, or one area, can compensate for another in which you have scored poorly. As candidates typically find the SBA questions harder to score well in, it is very important that, in the SAQ paper, they do not aim merely for the pass mark of 12 to16 out of 20. By thinking broadly and completely, it is possible to achieve a score of 16 or more. These additional marks will improve the total score should they perform poorly in the SBA section. The maximum score possible is 660 marks—the SAQ paper has 240 marks and the MCQ/SBA paper has 420 marks available. The scores from each paper are converted to a percentage, then summed. This means both the MCQ/SBA and the SAQ papers have equal weighting. The pass mark is set by the examiners using modified Angoff referencing which, to allow for exam reliability, is subsequently reduced by one standard error of the mean (SEM) to give the pass mark. Therefore, candidates who fail by only 1% have, in fact, significantly underperformed when compared to the actual pass mark and to the cohort of candidates as a whole.

Table 8.1 Annex C: knowledge competencies listed for the regional unit of training

Knowledge competence	Description	Assessment methods
RA_IK_01	Demonstrates understanding of basic sciences as applied to all regional anaesthesia blocks.	A, C, D, E
RA_IK_02	Knows advantages and disadvantages, techniques and complications of a variety of blocks (including those used in chronic pain conditions).	A, C, D, E
RA_IK_03	Demonstrates understanding in the choice of local anaesthetic agents, opioids, use of additives, and techniques of administration.	A, C, D, E

Reproduced with permission from the Royal College of Anaesthetists

MCQ section

The MCQ/SBA paper has 90 questions to be answered within three hours. Pressure of time is not usually a problem in this paper, so remain calm and read the instructions and the questions slowly and deliberately. It is better to go through the paper once, thoroughly, rather than rushing through it the first time before returning to check, change, and double check (and perhaps change again) your original answers. Doing so will leave you confused and full of self doubt. While continuing to read the questions thoroughly and taking your time, it should also be said that your first conclusion as to whether a question is true or false is usually correct. You have studied the length and breadth of the curriculum in preparation for this exam so you should trust yourself, trust that your knowledge is complete, and that if a statement is made of which you have never heard anything before, it is unlikely to be true.

The categories of questions in this section of the exam changed to reflect the units of training more closely and came into effect from August 2014. The RCoA website will have up-to-date information about the content of the exam as well as many other useful resources to download and use in candidates' preparation. This change to the source topics of the questions reflects the importance of each of the units of training at Intermediate Level. Candidates should be cognizant of the fact that of those who fail, many have little or no experience in particular clinical areas and underestimate the importance and prevalence of specialist units of training in the exam, particularly anaesthesia for cardiothoracic surgery, neurosurgery, and paediatrics. The advice in the Chairman's report is that all candidates should visit and experience taster days in these clinical areas if they have not completed the unit of training before sitting the Final exam.

The first 60 true/false MCQs consist of:

- 20 in advanced sciences to underpin anaesthetic practice
- 20 from the general duties' units of training
- 17 from the specialist (mandatory) units of training
- 3 from the optional units of training.

One mark is awarded for each correct answer in the true/false section. There is no negative marking, so all five parts of every question should be answered.

There are 30 SBA questions consisting of:

- 15 from the general duties' units of training
- 15 from the specialist (mandatory) units of training.

Four marks are awarded for each correct question in the SBA section. This reflects the fact that four answers have been eliminated in the course of choosing the best answer. Candidates often state this is an unfair 'all or nothing' way to mark these questions. They commonly report finding it difficult to choose between the final two options and receive no credit for eliminating three of the options. This is true. However, each time your choice is narrowed down to two options, there is a 50% chance that *anyone* would choose the correct one at random. Hopefully, with your extensive preparation, you will be significantly more likely to choose the correct one. The realistic way to look at this is that you will get some individual questions correct and some incorrect. When taken in the context of 30 questions, you should easily be able to get more than 15 (half of them) correct.

Read the questions accurately

This applies to all parts of every exam and is worth repeating. You *must* read the questions properly if you are to have a chance of answering them correctly. Continually, in practice sessions, candidates realize their mistakes and say 'Oh, I thought it said . . .' or, more honestly, 'I read it as saying . . .'. Remember, there is no time pressure in this paper. Take your time to read and understand each question properly.

Some candidates also fall into the trap of 'recognizing' the first part of a question that they have seen before. They assume the latter part of the question is identical too, and do not bother to finish reading it, or only skim over it quickly. They go straight to the answers and choose the option they remember being correct the first time without too much consideration as to whether it is still correct in view of the question now being asked. In other questions, the candidate will see the correct drug or physiological value in the answer but fail to notice whether the dose or units are correct, too. This is an easy way to throw away marks. You must not assume anything or take short cuts through the question when you see what you think is the correct answer listed. Questions can, and do, change subtly between sittings of the exam and a single word substitution may alter the thrust of the question entirely. Read the whole question carefully and think about what you are being asked.

When examiners construct new questions for this paper, particular attention is paid to the wording in an attempt to make the question clear and devoid of ambiguity. There are no words used by accident; each has been carefully considered. Pay close attention to the words used and their meaning.

For the Final exam, 'buzz words' in the questions may inform the answer. Words such as 'always' and 'never' are black and white options. 'Always' in the question is usually a true statement unless you can think of *any* instance where or when the action does not occur. If you see 'never', the statement is likely to be false. Bear in mind it is difficult to write a question confidently knowing that X *never* occurs; it takes a great deal of literature searching to confirm that is indeed the case, and such questions will become inaccurate and redundant if and when a case report detailing X crops up somewhere in the world. 'Softer' statements are common. Words such as 'usually', 'commonly', 'can', and 'may' indicate an action occurring with differing degrees of frequency. They 'usually' indicate the statement is true. Try to notice these 'buzz words' in the next few paragraphs.

As for any true/false MCQ paper, my advice is always to fill in the answer grid as you progress through the paper, question by question. Stop to check, after every question, that the following one is lined up correctly and that you have not missed out any rows or answered two questions in the same row. Doing this will double check your alignment and pick up any mistakes contemporaneously, preventing confusion at a later stage. This sounds incredibly obvious but such basic errors continue to occur regularly.

Please *avoid* writing all your answers on the question paper and transferring them all over to the answer grid in one go, at the end of the exam. There are several reasons for this advice. Firstly, if one answer is placed in the incorrect row, so too will all subsequent answers be in the wrong place. It is bad enough failing an exam, but failing due to such a silly mistake is even worse. Secondly, at the end of the exam you may be rushing or even be running out of time to transfer all the answers over. Rushing at this stage increases the chance of transcription errors. The most important reason to avoid this transferring technique is that it forces you to look again at your answer to each question. You will do so quickly to confirm your original answer and, in your haste, will misread and misunderstand questions. You will then decide to change your answer at the last minute—that answer you arrived at slowly and deliberately first time through. Aghast at how you could have managed to get it so wrong the first time, you will lose confidence in the rest of your decisions and will try to go over all your answers again, as you are transferring them, as the clock is ticking. You will become panicked and flustered and prone to errors. In my opinion, this is a recipe for disaster.

SBA section

The SBAs are not popular with exam candidates. There is a general consensus that they are unfair, that it is impossible to choose the correct 'best' answer as this can be a matter of opinion, and that these questions are the reason candidates fail the exam. These comments are not however supported by exam success data; the pass rate for this paper was consistent, at around 70%, before and after the introduction of the SBA component in September 2011. The fact remains that candidates who fail this part of the exam have a gap somewhere in their knowledge. The SBAs are here to stay, at present, so we should decide the best way to tackle them in advance of the exam.

I believe the concept behind the SBAs is misunderstood by candidates. When I ask candidates to write an SBA question, they inevitably provide a five-part, A to E, multiple choice question, where there is only one correct answer. The finer points of SBA questions are lost among quickly written revision aids containing what the authors believe to be exam-standard questions, when often they are not. Further, because SBAs are a new element to the FRCA, there is a limited bank of questions that the RCoA can publicize. Both these factors make practice at these questions difficult.

Questions for the exam itself are written to exacting standards and follow a set format. Rather than testing simple factual knowledge, SBAs test deduction, critical appraisal, and balancing of risks in an often complex clinical setting. Their aim is to assess *application* of important clinical knowledge within a *specific clinical context*, rather than the recall of isolated facts. The SBAs are written very precisely to a template containing many rules. Each question will focus on an important concept that would be encountered in clinical practice, as opposed to trivial topics or minor peculiarities. The stem, or introduction, consists of a vignette of clinical or laboratory information which can be up to 60 words in length. This will be followed by a short lead-in to the choice of the best answer. The lead-in should be a simple, direct question answerable by applying knowledge and information presented in the stem. The five options are short and should each relate to a single factor only. There should be no double options; for example, 'Do X because of Y' should instead be 'Do X'.

Questions are rigorously tested by a generic cohort of examiners rather than specialists in the relevant fields. They are modified to avoid ambiguity, remove confusing factors, and to ensure they are as clear as possible.

In SBA questions, all five answers will be plausible; several may also be possible; more than one or two answers may be correct or acceptable; but one option will be better than the others, and that is the answer. It is often the case that three options can be clearly eliminated and it is difficult to decide between the remaining two. There may be debate around the 'best' answers; some having a degree of subjectivity, and others reflecting true variations between the varied practice of different clinicians. At times, not all the examiners will agree on what the best answer ought to be. This makes it difficult for trainers and candidates to predict what, specifically, makes the best answer better than the others. The RCoA look for the answer that they would expect to receive from a competent higher trainee in anaesthesia (that is, one at the beginning of ST5 who is practicing safely and who errs on the side of caution). Notably, the best answer is not that given by a consultant with a niche role in the particular clinical area. It is also not the answer given by a very experienced consultant who may know 'what works for me' and will draw on their lengthy experience to aid clinical decision making.

When two correct options remain, candidates should choose the simplest one, the least invasive one, the one with the lowest risk to the patient, the safest one. Choose the right answer and you receive four marks, but choose the wrong one and you gain zero marks. In these circumstances, where you must choose between the final two, you would expect anyone to be correct 50% of the time and, following months of studying, you should be correct more than 50% of the time. Let us say you guess correctly 60% of the time. This means that for every ten questions you could not work out the best answer and have guessed, you would score 24 out of 40. This is a mark consistent with passing the paper. Even if you only guess correctly 50% of the time, you will still score 20 out of 40. All scores are summed. Do not blame the SBAs for making you fail the exam. It is *your* exam to pass or fail.

The first rule of answering these questions is to find your correct answer within the list of five options. To do so, it is important not to colour your judgement by what you see listed there, because all the options may sound reasonable. My advice is to firstly *cover over all five options* to the question. Next, read the stem and the lead-in. Then STOP. Do not look at the options yet. Stop and think about the question, note the specific wording, decide what it is asking, and think about what you would actually do in your clinical practice when faced with this scenario. SBA questions are often written subsequent to real-life clinical dilemmas. If you do not know what you would do, think who you would ask to help you and what kind of help you would require. Do you need help to decide between two options? Do you need help with a specific skill only? Or do you need help with the decision making? In case of the latter, try to imagine what your senior colleague would advise you to do if you telephoned him or her with this scenario. What if he or she were a Final examiner? What would he or she suggest you do? Once you have formulated what you believe to be the answer, only then uncover the options. If the answer you have arrived at is there, excellent! This is the one to select. Do not be tempted to change your mind to any of the distracters (incorrect answers). Congratulate yourself on having the self discipline to cover the answers while you stop and think, because this is difficult to do.

If your answer is not listed, then you have to use a different strategy. Try to eliminate as many wrong answers as you can. If you can eliminate four, then that is fantastic. If, however, you can only eliminate three, you must apply the 'best guess' strategy to the remaining two answers, as detailed earlier in this chapter.

Remember to think of the patient safety initiative—'Stop before you block'—introduced to prevent inadvertent wrong-sided placement of peripheral nerve blocks. This asks you to stop and recheck the side, needle poised, immediately prior to its insertion into the skin. Apply the same technique in this paper. Immediately before reading the question, stop and cover the answers. You must 'Stop before you (mentally) block'.

Since August 2014, a pass in the written part of the Final exam (MCQ/SBA and SAQ papers) is valid for three years, taken to the date of the SOE applied for. However, my advice would be to take the SOE as soon as possible after passing the written paper. Keep some exam focus and momentum going in your life, even if it is the last thing you feel like doing. Often, candidates feel they have to prioritize their time to other areas of their lives after the commitment of studying for the written paper but, in my experience, candidates who delay taking the SOE always regret doing so, and state they wish they had carried on to take it straight away.

There is no perfect time to sit exams; the best time is now. Do it. Make a huge effort and do it well, first time round, and minimize the duration of its impact in your life.

CHAPTER 9

The Short Answer Question (SAQ) paper

CONTENTS

The Short Answer Question (SAQ) paper is the part of the exam where your score can depend on how well you present what you know. What you actually know is important, too, and the questions that candidates often fail due to lack of knowledge include anatomy, pharmacokinetics, and subspecialty areas such as paediatrics and cardiac anaesthesia. Clinically inexperienced candidates also fail to score maximum marks by providing a correct but very limited answer, where the common elements are known but the full breadth of knowledge is lacking. In Figure 9.1, the written content is correct but is far from complete, and is what I term a 'primary' answer. The candidate has also failed to consider the allocation of marks to each part of the question.

Other questions that candidates often fail require knowledge that they know well by this stage in training, but they have been unable to extract the *specific parts* of that knowledge required to answer the question. Past examples include oxygen therapy, massive haemorrhage, and anaesthetizing a patient with a fractured neck of femur. Questions on such poorly answered topics are modified and included in future papers.

If, as part of your answer, you mention tests that you would carry out, you must state the *reasons why* you are doing these tests. Foundation doctors may request 'routine bloods' but, for the Final FRCA exam, you will request a full blood count to check the platelet level before regional anaesthesia, the haemoglobin concentration before moderate or extensive surgery and the differential white cell count to help make your diagnosis.

The questions

- 12 compulsory questions in three hours, normally on the principles and practice of clinical anaesthesia.
- All 12 questions must be attempted; candidates will fail if one or more questions are not attempted.
- Questions in the wrong answer book will not normally be marked.

The 12 questions come directly from the Intermediate Training section of the 2010 Curriculum. There will be a question on each of the six essential units of training (obstetric anaesthesia, intensive care medicine, chronic pain, neuro-anaesthesia, cardio-thoracic anaesthesia, and paediatric anaesthesia). There will be four questions taken from the general units of training (or guidelines pertaining to practice in these areas) which include common surgical specialties, airway management, and resuscitation. The final two questions are derived from the optional units of training (vascular anaesthesia, plastic surgery, and ophthalmic anaesthesia).

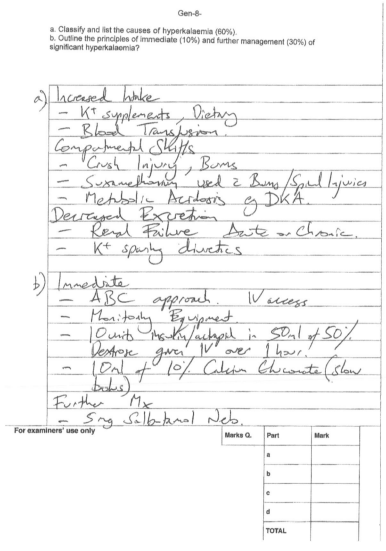

Gen-8-

a. Classify and list the causes of hyperkalaemia (60%).
b. Outline the principles of immediate (10%) and further management (30%) of significant hyperkalaemia?

Figure 9.1 Example of a 'primary' answer with correct but incomplete content.

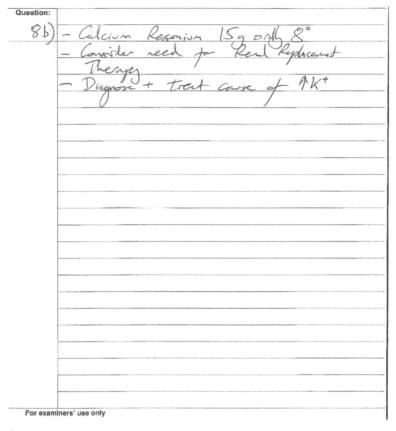

Question:

8b) – Calcium Resonium 15g orally 8°
    – Consider need for Renal Replacement
      Therapy
    – Diagnose + treat cause of ↑K⁺

For examiners' use only

Figure 9.1 Continued

The marking

- Each question is marked out of 20. The pass mark for each question is determined by the examiners collectively using a modified Angoff reference method.
- The pass marks for the 12 questions are summed to give a total mark for the paper. To allow for exam reliability, this is then reduced by 1 × SEM to give the pass mark.
- The pass mark is the sum of the percentage pass marks of the MCQ and SAQ papers.
- The pass mark for each paper will be calculated as a percentage and rounded down to two decimal places.
- The resultant pass marks for each paper are added together and the combined percentage score rounded down to one decimal place.

The questions are graded easy, moderate, or difficult at the paper setting, and the pass mark for each question can range from 10–16 out of 20. There are no 'sudden death' questions or marks deducted for incorrect statements, so do not cross out anything that you have written including your rough notes. Candidates should attain every mark possible with their answer, striving for it to be as good as possible, rather than just aiming to achieve the pass mark. No half marks are awarded. Drugs should be accompanied by the appropriate dose (mg/kg) and it is preferable to use generic names.

The score from this paper is summed with that achieved in the MCQ/SBA paper which means that any additional marks gained here will help to prop up a poorer score on those parts of the paper which candidates traditionally find more difficult.

Time management

Candidates are continually caught out by poor time management in this paper; 12 questions are to be answered in three hours. The time allocation for each question must be adhered to strictly. It can be difficult to stop writing when you still have more to say, but stop you must. You can always return to write more if you have spare time at the end, but if you even spend 90 seconds too long on each of the first 11 questions, you will have no time left to attempt question 12. This is devastating, as all questions must be attempted in order to pass the paper. If taking more time over some questions leaves no time for another, you *will* fail the paper. This is an exhausting paper both mentally and physically, but you must focus on the time as well as the content.

The complete answers have been trialled by examiners at the RCoA to ensure each can be answered fully within 10 minutes, using only a single side of paper. Therefore, it is vital that your preparation includes time-based practice. In our local practice, the time allowed for each question is limited strictly to 12 minutes. This allows time for reading the paper at the start and thinking about your answers. Strict adherence to this rule will prevent you spending too long on questions where you know very little or indeed, know too much. In the latter instance, the temptation is to write down everything you know, taking additional time to do so. Beware, there are no extra marks available for additional information over and above that required to score the full 20 marks, even if your written content is correct. Marks are awarded strictly in line with the marking scheme (which reflects the distribution shown in the question) and are only awarded for facts which are on that marking scheme.

You should practise several SAQs together. Four questions per hour or six per ninety minutes will give you a feel for the intensity of the exam and the fatigue that develops during this paper. Practising 12 questions in three hours is worthwhile too, but I would not suggest doing this too close to the actual exam.

Handwriting and presentation

This paper is a test of conveying your knowledge clearly, concisely, and efficiently. To score points, the examiner must be able to read what you have written, so it is also very much a test of handwriting. We each think our own handwriting is easy to read, when in fact it can be very difficult to an unaccustomed eye. Have a colleague review one of your practice questions. Can they read it easily? Swap papers with another trainee preparing for the exam. Can you read their writing as easily as your own? Figure 9.2 is subjectively 'neat' writing but is still difficult for others to read.

Note the differences between British, European, Indian, or male and female handwriting. The examiners will each have a large pile of questions to mark, with all types of handwriting to decipher. Make sure yours is easy for them to read. Legibility itself will not get you any more marks per se but does mean you will not lose out on any you deserve, and you may be afforded the benefit of any doubt. Remember, the examiners do not receive payment to mark exam papers. Each examiner will mark two questions and usually has around 100 answers to mark and return within two weeks. This is clearly an onerous task and while examiners will make some effort to determine what has been written and be as fair as possible, poor handwriting can make a slow laborious process increasingly difficult. If your paper is presented neatly and clearly, the examiner

Gen-8-

a. Classify and list the causes of hyperkalaemia (60%).
b. Outline the principles of immediate (10%) and further management (30%) of significant hyperkalaemia?

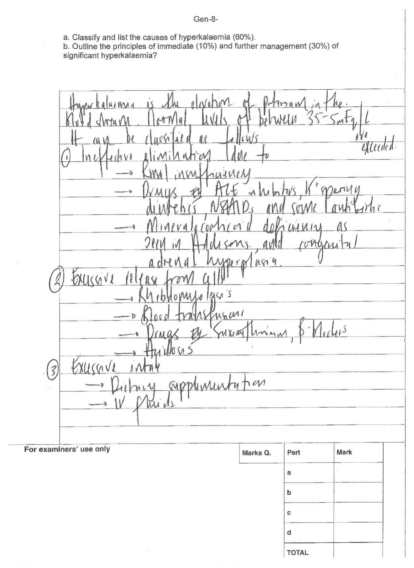

Figure 9.2 Example of 'neat' handwriting that is still difficult to read.

will be very happy. Marks are given for what is legible. No marks are withheld due to poor presentation alone but if the examiner cannot read it, then they cannot assess its merit.

In Figure 9.3, the answer appears to begin well, following the classification of the question. However, by part B and beyond, the presentation is very messy, sloppy, and difficult to make sense of. In part A, note that there are nine marks for 'patient considerations' (45%). This means that at least nine points of information must be made. This answer shows fewer than nine and only one mentions the patient's diabetes, and this in an inadequate and vague manner. What facts about his diabetes would you want to know? What is his definition of 'good' and what is your own?

Gen -11-

A 75 year old man with type 2 diabetes (tablet controlled) presents for elective inguinal hernia repair.
a) What are the patient (45%) and surgical (15%) factors at pre-op assessment that would make him suitable for day surgery.
b) What are the anaesthetic consideration (intra-op and post-op) in this case for day surgery (40%)

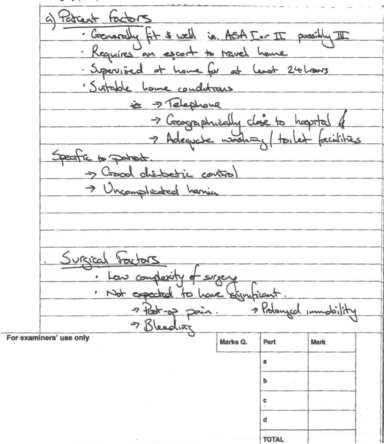

a) Patient factors
· Generally fit & well ie. ASA I or II possibly III
· Requires an escort to travel home
· Supervised at home for at least 24 hours
· Suitable home conditions
      ie → Telephone
         → Geographically close to hospital &
         → Adequate washing / toilet facilities
Specific to patient.
   → Good diabetic control
   → Uncomplicated hernia

· Surgical factors
   · Low complexity of surgery
   · Not expected to have Significant.
      → Post-op pain.   → Prolonged immobility
      → Bleeding

For examiners' use only

Marks Q.	Part	Mark
	a	
	b	
	c	
	d	
	TOTAL	

Figure 9.3 Example of messy presentation.

Pay attention to the basics, such as avoiding a blotchy pen, and try different pens to find one which enhances your writing. Figure 9.4 shows how, when using an ink pen, the ink soaks through the page distorting the answer on both sides.

In pursuit of clarity, many candidates resort to writing entirely in CAPITAL LETTERS. If this is truly the clearest way for you to write, then go ahead, but I try to discourage this practice as it is time-consuming and, more importantly, the shape of the word is lost. When reading suboptimal handwriting, we rely more on looking for words we might expect to see and the shape those words form. We then decide if we can recognize the word or phrase we are looking for within the written text. The height and shape of the component letters is an important form of pattern recognition and is best retained. Using full capitalization for titles, headings, and subheadings only, is a good compromise.

Question: b) Anaesthetic considerations

~~Pre-op~~ Intra-op

- Aim to limit post-operative nausea & vomiting
  - Limit opiate
    - → Use of simple analgesics
    - → Regional ~~[illegible]~~ anaesthesia where appropriate
    - → Ilioinguinal block.
  - Volatile free anaesthesia.
  - Screen for risk factors & give prophylaxis if required.
- Monitor blood glucose levels hourly
- Muscle relaxation may be required ~~for~~ to facilitate surgery

For examiners' use only

Question: Post-operative

- Rescue anti-emetics should be prescribed.
- Rescue analgesic.
- Appropriate discharge analgesic prescribed & available for patient to take home.
- Encourage early return to diet & recommencement of diabetic medication once eating & drinking
- Discharge criteria according to local protocol should be met prior to discharge.

For examiners' use only

Figure 9.3 Continued

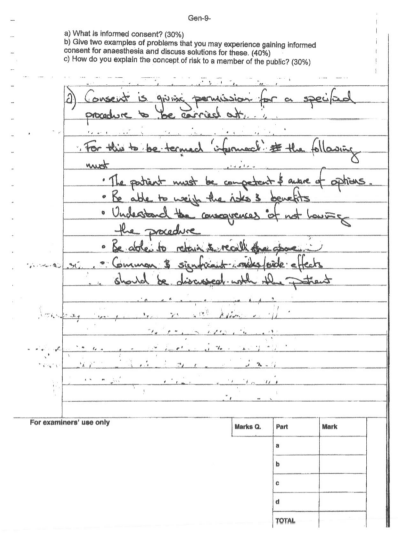

Gen-9-

a) What is informed consent? (30%)
b) Give two examples of problems that you may experience gaining informed consent for anaesthesia and discuss solutions for these. (40%)
c) How do you explain the concept of risk to a member of the public? (30%)

a) Consent is giving permission for a specified procedure to be carried out.

For this to be termed 'informed' the following must
• The patient must be competent & aware of options.
• Be able to weigh the risks & benefits
• Understand the consequences of not having the procedure
• Be able to retain & recall the above
• Common & significant risks/side effects should be discussed with the patient

For examiners' use only		Marks Q.	Part	Mark
			a	
			b	
			c	
			d	
			TOTAL	

Figure 9.4 Avoid using ink that can soak through the page.

You should space out your answer (see Figure 9.5). There is no shortage of pages in the exam booklets and if you still need more, additional pages can be clipped in. Spacing out your answer makes it clearer (especially if your writing is untidy) and leaves room for you to add anything else you remember later on without cramming it in between what is already written, or into the bottom corner of the page, or in a completely separate area with directions for the examiner to follow to find it.

Do not write in the bottom section of each page labelled 'examiner's use only'. Not only will this annoy the examiner, there is a risk that anything written there will be disregarded (see Figure 9.6).

To present your knowledge clearly, it should not be wrapped up in prose. This paper is not a test of the English language, grammar, sentence structure, or poetic ability. There are no marks

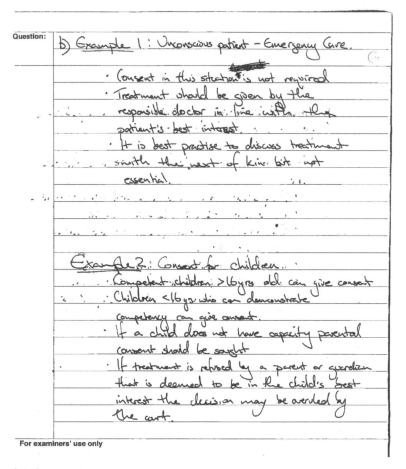

Question:

b) Example 1: Unconscious patient - Emergency Care.

· Consent in this situation is not required
· Treatment should be given by the
  responsible doctor in line with the
  patient's best interest.
· It is best practise to discuss treatment
  with the next of kin but not
  essential.

Example 2: Consent for children.
· Competent children >16yrs old can give consent
· Children <16yrs who can demonstrate
  competency can give consent.
· If a child does not have capacity parental
  consent should be sought
· If treatment is refused by a parent or guardian
  that is deemed to be in the child's best
  interest the decision may be overuled by
  the court.

For examiners' use only

Figure 9.4 Continued

available for flowery language or any words superfluous to the facts. Do not copy out the question at the top of the page. There is no need to construct a general, introductory sentence. The questions should be answered using short, bullet-pointed factual statements as far as possible. Lists should run vertically, making them easy to read at a glance. Large answers should be classified (and I will discuss this in more detail). Using diagrams can be a good, fast way to show what you mean. Diagrams should be titled and large, neat, and clearly labelled. Lines should be drawn straight and do try to avoid scribbling out errors. Similarly, graphs need titles and straight axes which are each labelled with the correct units of measurement. Look back at the graphs shown in Chapters 1 and 2.

Classification

Classification of your answer is important for many reasons. It is absolutely essential for questions covering a large topic or period, for example: 'Describe the peri-operative management of [any large case]' or 'How may we prevent post-operative nausea and vomiting?'. Increasingly, a

Intensive Care –4–

List the indications (15%), contra-indications (25%), benefits (20%) and complications (40%) of percutaneous tracheostomy on the intensive care unit.

INDICATIONS : Need for prolonged mechanical ventilation
Airway obstruction – neoplasm
– vocal cord palsy
– laryngeal trauma
– oedema
Need for pulmonary toilet – inadequate cough
– aspiration
Comfort of patient
Prevent complications of long-term trans-laryngeal intubation.

CONTRA-INDICATIONS
– Obesity/Short neck with poor landmarks
– Coagulopathy
– Infection at site of proposed incision.

BENEFITS
– Decreased bleeding risk
– Avoids transfer of critically ill patient
– Improved wound healing.

For examiners' use only	Marks Q.	Part	Mark
		a	
		b	
		c	
		d	
		TOTAL	

Figure 9.5 Example of classification of questions being followed, using a spacious layout.

degree of classification is built into the question, so look out for such clues to help structure your answer.

By classifying your answer, you provide a framework for it. You have the basics defined and can then expand your answer, hanging further information around it as appropriate. Your classification will act as an *aide-mémoir* for you, helping to ensure you answer all aspects of the question, rather than just the obvious basics. Classification immediately shows you to be organized in your thought processes and systematic in your approach, both to the answer and, by inference, as you would be in the clinical situation. This makes a good impression with the examiner.

Classification provides you with convenient subheadings to your answer. You can space these out and add to them later if need be. This will be easier to do if you make your lists run vertically.

Intensive Care -2-

A 70kg, 30 year old man presents with burns following a house fire. The burns are confined to his torso and upper limbs, but exclude his head and neck.

a) State the Parkland formula used for burns fluid resuscitation? (10%)
b) His burns are estimated at 40% of his body surface area. Using the Parkland formula, what volume of fluid will he require in the first 8 hours after injury? (10%)
c) What additional fluids in excess of the volume predicted in (b) might he require and why? (20%)
d) What investigations (40%) and monitoring (20%) are required in the first 24 hours? Please state reasons for each.

a) The Parkland formula is used to calculate the amount of fluid required during the resuscitation of patients with burns based on their bodyweight and % burn area.

Fluids required in the first 24 hours is equal to weight in kilograms multiplied by the % surface area of the burn multiplied by 4.

b) 40 × 4 × 70 = 11200
   5600 ml in first 4 hours

c) The patient may require further fluids including blood - if they are bleeding or coagulation factors live via FFP + cryoprecipitate. Platelets if platelets are low

d) Investigations may include a full blood count as patients can become anaemic or thrombocytopenic. U+E's to monitor K+ in particular as K+ can rise. Also to monitor for AKI. Monitoring of urine output. Check Mg/PO4 as they can vary after burns. Check CK + myoglobin. Check coag
   Monitor HR, BP, SpO2, ABG's.
   ECG
   CXR

For examiners' use only
CO lamb

Marks Q.	Part	Mark
	a	
	b	
	c	
	d	
	TOTAL	

Figure 9.6 Avoid breaching the examiner's space.

There are a few classification systems that can be applied to many questions. I have included some, as examples, but this list is not exhaustive and you may have some of your own.

Example 1: Management of anaesthetic for . . . any surgical problem

a. Pre-operative considerations
b. Induction plan
c. Intra-operative course
d. Post-operative plan
e. Specific issues unique to the subject in question

This plan will allow you to answer a question on a surgical procedure which is unfamiliar to you. Questions with unusual surgical procedures are passed by only a small percentage of candidates. Regardless of the procedure, all patients presenting for surgery can be managed on this time-based, progressive approach, which is familiar to all anaesthetists. By following it, you will usually find you are able to write enough to pass the question, as long as you do not panic and think 'I've never heard of this, have never seen it, and cannot answer it' and either have a meltdown or give up without making an attempt. Think of major cases you *have* done or seen and what they involved. Then transfer the parts of that knowledge that could be applicable to this lesser known case. Is massive haemorrhage a risk? Is it a particularly lengthy case? What position must the patient adopt? Does the surgeon have any specific requirements (paralysis, hypotension, pro-coagulants)? State that you would liaise with the surgeon about the planned procedure and address any outstanding queries you have at the theatre huddle prior to starting the case—just as you would do in reality.

Example 2: Describe the anatomy of . . . any structure

Anatomical descriptions should include the relevant information from this list.

a. Boundaries: superior, inferior, lateral, medial, posterior, and anterior
b. Relations: superior, inferior, lateral, medial, posterior, and anterior
c. Contents
d. Shape
e. Blood supply
f. Nerve supply
g. Special features

A drawing may also be helpful (as already stated) and can convey information at a glance which may take a few sentences to write out. Diagrams are particularly helpful if your handwriting is poor.

See Figure 9.7 and compare the ways in which the candidates have tackled a question on the anatomy of the epidural space. Which one would you find easiest to mark? Which one clearly shows the candidate knows the facts required?

Example 3: What are the complications of . . . any procedure

a. Immediate
b. Early
c. Late

Or

a. Common
b. Rare
c. Very rare

You should provide some estimate of what you mean by 'rare' and 'very rare'. Give an occurrence rate, such as occurring in 1% of cases. You can explain this to the patient as being 1 in 100 cases or equivalent to someone in a small village being affected.

Example 4: What are the causes of . . . any symptom/sign/problem

a. Physiological (Cushings or stress response, homeostatic mechanism)
b. Pathological (inflammatory, neoplastic, autoimmune, infective)
c. Pharmacological (iatrogenic, anaphylactoid, anaphylactic, idiosyncratic reactions, expected side-effects)

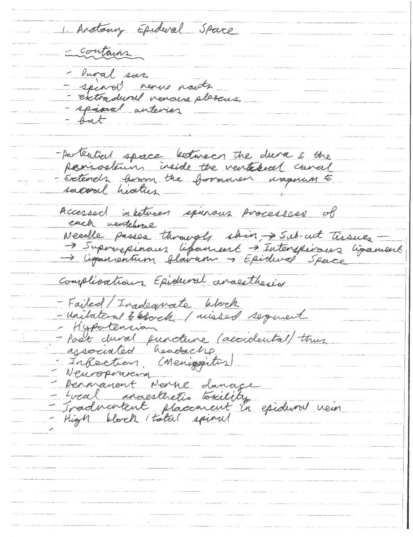

1. Anatomy Epidural Space

  — contains

    - Dural sac
    - spinal nerve roots
    - extradural venous plexus
    - spinal arteries
    - fat

    - potential space between the dura & the periosteum inside the vertebral canal
    - Extends from the foramen magnum to sacral hiatus

    Accessed in between spinous processes of each vertebra
    Needle passes through skin → Sub-cut Tissues → Supraspinous ligament → Interspinous ligament → Ligamentum flavum → Epidural Space

    Complications Epidural anaesthesia

    - Failed / Inadequate block
    - unilateral block / missed segment
    - Hypotension
    - Post dural puncture (accidental) thus associated headache
    - Infection (Meningitis)
    - Neuropraxia
    - Permanent nerve damage
    - Local anaesthetic toxicity
    - Inadvertent placement in epidural vein
    - High block / total spinal
    -

Figure 9.7 Examples of two alternative ways of tackling a question.

Or

a. Patient-related causes
b. Anaesthetic-related causes
c. Surgical causes
d. 'Other' causes (which leave a catch-all option for later additions)

Or

a. Congenital
   i. Inherited
  ii. Sporadic

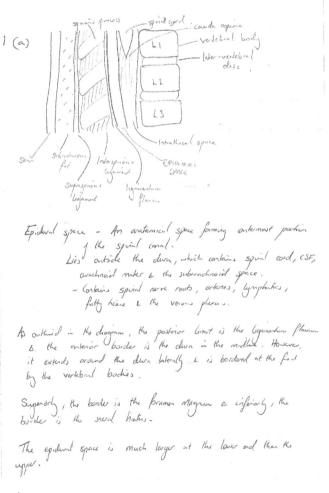

1 (a)

Epidural space – An anatomical space forming outermost portion of the spinal canal.
Lies outside the dura, which contains spinal cord, CSF, arachnoid mater & the subarachnoid space.
– Contains spinal nerve roots, arteries, lymphatics, fatty tissue & the venous plexus.

As outlined in the diagram, the posterior limit is the ligamentum flavum & the anterior border is the dura in the midline. However, it extends around the dura laterally & is bordered at the front by the vertebral bodies.

Superiorly, the border is the foramen magnum & inferiorly, the border is the sacral hiatus.

The epidural space is much larger at the lower end than the upper.

Figure 9.7 Continued

b. Acquired
  i. Infective
  ii. Neoplastic
  iii. Autoimmune
  iv. Inflammatory
  v. Drug-induced
  vi. Iatrogenic

Example 5: How would you perform . . . any block

a. Pre-operative anaesthetic assessment of patient
b. Discussion of block and other options; consent
c. Preparation of anaesthetic room (equipment, drugs, assistance, IV access, monitors)
d. Identify landmarks

e. Prepare sterile field

f. Use ultrasound, if appropriate

g. Type of needle and nerve stimulator

h. Injectate choice

i. Performing the block

This last example shows how, if asked to describe a block you are not familiar with, a large part of the question is about the process common to all types of blocks and familiar to all anaesthetists. Therefore, do not panic that you do not know the answer. Think about what you do know about nerve blocks and apply it to this situation.

Some specifics

There is a 'driving test' element to this paper in that you must remember to deliberately state all the basic things that you or your anaesthetic assistant do automatically. This includes attaching monitors, preparing equipment, and administering oxygen. Remember to state that you have checked the machine and established IV access and have emergency drugs available. If it is not written down, it cannot be assumed that it has been done, and no marks can be awarded.

Targetting your revision

There is an element of making your own luck in exams. The more you have learned and practised, the luckier you will be with the range of questions that present themselves in your exam. Question spotting alone is a very high-risk strategy on which to base your studying and is not recommended. Although the same questions do appear repeatedly in exams, they are usually modified, to a greater or lesser extent, and the emphasis may be different. As well as reading the question accurately, you must ensure you answer the question asked. For example, a paediatric question could begin with 'A six-year-old child presents for day-case circumcision' and may continue thus:

a. Outline the requirements for same-day discharge. (30%)

b. Describe the options for analgesia. (30%)

c. List the components of EMLA cream. (15%)

d. What are the advantages and disadvantages of using EMLA? (15%)

Or may ask instead:

a. What are the anaesthetic considerations in this patient? (40%)

b. List the criteria for admission post-operatively. (25%)

c. He is accompanied by his maternal grandparents with whom he lives. Discuss the issue of consent for anaesthesia. (35%)

These two questions will clearly require two very different answers. Do not fall into the trap of writing all you know about paediatrics and day surgery in the hope that you will score some marks. Further there is no time to do this so you must target your answer to that which is asked.

You should cover the broad base of the curriculum but, in addition, certain areas can be identified as being more likely to appear in any exam and can be targetted for extra, specific studying. The more you do this, the more you will be rewarded and the luckier you will become.

Think of the 12 questions you would least like to see when you turn over the question paper. Make a note of them. Now go and learn about each of these topics in turn. Next, make up a question about each topic and answer it within 12 minutes. If your answer is not as good as you had hoped, go back and decide what is missing. Correct it. Improve it. Write it out again, and again, and again if need be. When that question appears in the exam, you will feel lucky that a topic you studied so well has been asked, will you not? You have made your own luck. Now do the same process with the next topic on your list.

Questions pertaining to current or recent guidelines are increasing in prevalence. National or international guidelines will be referred to rather than local, regional publications or policies in devolved nations. Examples include the World Health Organization (Surgical Checklist), Medical Royal Colleges, the Association of Anaesthetists of Great Britain and Ireland ('glossies'), and the General Medical Council's pamphlet for doctors pertaining to good practice and child protection. Questions are based on the units of training in the 2010 Curriculum which is continually being updated. Newer, more recently incorporated areas will be used in due course for question development and include quality improvement and anaesthesia for endovascular procedures.

As clinical practice evolves, so too will the questions change to reflect this. Drug eluting stents, newer anticoagulants, the increase in interventional radiology, and cardiopulmonary exercise testing will all lead to questions being developed to cover these areas.

Read the question carefully

It is usually the case that candidates who fail to score well on basic questions and routine topics which are commonly asked, do so because they misread or misinterpret the question. There is little to say about misreading the question other than *read the question carefully*, then read it again to confirm what you think it asks. It is often reported by the Chairman in his report that the actual question asked was not answered specifically. Many give good generalized accounts of the subject in question without focussing in on the component parts and details specifically asked for.

Misinterpretation, or setting off at a tangent to the actual answer required, is a common reason for candidates to fail a question. This often happens with large, wide-ranging clinical scenarios about common surgical problems. Past questions asking about day-case anaesthesia for a diabetic patient having an eye operation and a frail patient with a fractured neck of femur presenting for surgery have had poor (<50%) pass rates due to candidates not answering the specific question asked. One way to avoid this is to read the question accurately (much thought is put into the wording of each question to ensure clarity and avoid ambiguity), read your answer, then read the question again and decide if your answer satisfies the question.

Another useful technique is to write your answer, then cover up the question, and read your answer in isolation. Can you tell from your answer what specifics the question asked for? Could your answer apply to *any* day-case procedure or *any* frail patient having *any* operation? If the latter is true, you have not answered the question asked and, even if what you have written is true, it will not score points if it does not include the answers on the examiner's ideal answer template.

Many questions include phrases such as 'What are the considerations . . .' or 'What are the principles . . .' regarding anaesthesia for different types of surgery. These questions do not require an account of the routine practice of general anaesthesia. They are asking 'What are your *specific* concerns and requirements for *this* case? Why is it different? What would you tell a junior to watch out for? Which parts of the operation causes particular problems? What is complicated about this case?'

Questions with 'What are the specific concerns . . .' or 'What are the anaesthetic issues regarding [a child/a diabetic/eye surgery/day surgery/etc.]' are often interpreted by candidates as 'Tell me all you know about . . .' and they can easily spend the whole time writing about a standard pre-operative assessment, general day-case criteria, or about paediatric weights, endotracheal tube sizes, and drug doses. These candidates fail to gain many of the marks available. What these questions are asking is 'What is different about this case?' when compared, for instance, to standard general anaesthesia for varicose vein surgery or an appendicectomy.

The meanings of some verbs used frequently in questions are outlined as follows:

List: make a list—bullet-pointed but not necessarily single words. Little or no additional information is required but can be expanded to show understanding.

Outline: also a list, plus a sentence or two of additional information about the basic features of each item on the list.

Describe: a fuller account of what is happening. 'Describe the anaesthetic techniques' means 'tell me what you would *do* to anaesthetize the patient'. Do not obscure this answer with 'Trained assistant, tipping trolley . . .'. It means '*do*' or '*state*', so proceed to the anaesthetic plan without delay.

Define: write the standard definition; for example, the definition of post-partum haemorrhage, chronic regional pain syndromes (CRPS) I and II.

Compare: examine two or more items through argument. This can be answered using a table to show advantages and disadvantages of each subject.

Classify: arrange in or assign to categories. Headings and subheadings are useful here.

Discuss: talk about. Think about in being in the coffee room, discussing your next case.

Principles: general rules or laws relevant to the matter in question. They are non-specific and are not tasks.

Common introductions to questions are: 'What is the *significance of* . . .' (means, why is it important?) and 'What are the *problems with* . . .' (means, why is it difficult?).

While reading the question, attention should also be paid to the breakdown of the question and the proportionate allocation of marks within it. The questions are split into two to four component parts, each with an allocated percentage of the total 20 marks available. A part worth 50% (ten marks) will require ten points or ten facts, at least, to score ten points. There may be 15 options on the answer sheet and ten marks will be awarded if any ten of the listed 15 are provided. You should plan to spend about half of the time on this part, which is around six minutes. Be aware that if you only write three or four reasons, you will score a maximum of three or four marks out of a possible ten. Ensure you write enough to be able to score all of the marks.

Similarly, if a component part of a question is worth 10% (only two marks), do not spend too long thinking about the answer if you are unsure. Alternatively, if you do know lots about that component, only write what is asked for. Remember, there will be no more than two marks available, no matter how much you write, no matter how correct it is. Do not waste precious time on these smaller value questions.

At the time of writing, the RCoA changed from annotating the SAQ component parts with percentages of the total to now stating the actual number of marks available for each part.

In summary

1 Strict timing is non-negotiable.
2 Write legibly.
3 Write more than only the obvious.
4 Practise writing out your answers within the time allowed.
5 Read the questions accurately and answer the questions asked.
6 Classify your answers for clarity and as a memory aid.
7 Use lists, bullet points, and diagrams.

CHAPTER 10

The Structured Oral Exams (SOEs)

CONTENTS

Preparation: if racing hurdles . . . practice hurdles!

You would think it crazy if someone training to run a marathon did all their training on a bicycle, planning only to run on race day. This statement sounds obvious but I never fail to be amazed at the number of people who prepare for the SOE by 'doing a bit more reading', or 'talking it through themselves', or 'talking to their cat'. The viva is the most dreaded part of any exam. Likewise, viva practice is also much maligned and is completely avoided by some candidates. This is short-sighted and reduces the chance of passing the exam.

We discussed in Chapter 9 that the best way to study for the SAQ paper is to practise timed SAQs in an environment as close as possible to that in the exam. Try to recreate this for the viva section, too. You should not need to acquire more knowledge; having passed the written papers you have enough knowledge to pass the vivas *if* you learn to present it clearly and concisely. While practising speaking aloud to yourself is helpful and allows you to plan how you may begin to answer questions, it is no substitute for sitting down with a senior, feeling the anxiety build, and tackling random questions as they are asked.

Viva practice *is* uncomfortable and it is unpleasant to put yourself through it. Do remember though that those senior to you have all been there, too. Many of us can remember the feelings experienced and of being under such pressure. Do not worry about looking stupid or losing face. The people you work with each day already know your capabilities and limitations and they will not think any less of you as a doctor. Viva performance is distinct from clinical practice and there are many good doctors who perform badly in oral exams for one reason or another (but usually because they have not practised). It is not easy, but then nothing worthwhile is easy. If the exam was easy there would be no accolade in passing it; and everyone would succeed.

You should have lots and lots of viva practice. Try to have at least one formal viva per day, and more if you can manage. You should actively seek out individuals in your department and ask them to viva you. You should arrange a time and place in advance; most of us like to prepare or at least think about what we are going to ask you and will not appreciate an impromptu 'Can I have a viva now?' request. You may have to fit these in before a late shift or in the morning after a night shift. You should arrange several during your days off. This is the best use of your time for these weeks leading up to the actual day of the SOE.

This preparation not only allows you to practise and perfect the words you will say, it also allows you to identify gaps in your knowledge. The more practice you have, the more subjects you will cover. You will undoubtedly uncover areas in which you need to improve and will still have time to remedy them. Perhaps a question will be asked from a different angle, with an emphasis on one element you had not previously considered. Perhaps, simply, areas where your knowledge is lacking will be discovered—in time! It is far better to perform poorly, make mistakes, have your mind go blank, and realize you know nothing about the topic in question *before* the actual exam. Remember, there is no charge for making mistakes in practice and it does not count as an attempt at the exam. Aim to make all your mistakes during practice.

Viva practice has many advantages. Most importantly, familiarity reduces anxiety. The more you have practised anticipating, waiting, then sitting down with stern, stony faced consultants, the more you will get used to this situation and the less anxious you will feel. It follows that you should approach the most intimidating people you know and ask them for viva practice. This may be the last thing you want to do but it will pay dividends come exam day.

You should have a realistic environment in which to practise speaking. Even the most knowledgeable candidates present their answers in a disorganized and random fashion if they have not prepared their delivery in advance. Practising how you will speak makes you think about what you will say, and provides an opportunity to order your thoughts and consider how best to present them in a logical manner. Your speech should reflect your experience and be delivered in a fluid, calm manner. You are being assessed as a mature trainee, about to enter the final stages of training. The final viva is the last major hurdle to be overcome and the examiner needs to see that you are a confident, credible clinician who is aware of various options available and who can make informed and balanced decisions on a patient by patient basis. You can practise adopting this persona at work each day, when you consider and discuss a case with the consultant or when speaking with colleagues in the coffee room as they enquire as to what you have on your list today. Speak as if you had a novice anaesthetist working with you, continually asking why you are doing things a certain way, asking what you have taken into consideration, asking why other doctors do it differently, and so on. This makes your explanations sound real and conveys an aura of experience; you have been in these situations before and have made decisions competently.

Viva practice provides an opportunity for a senior colleague to give you feedback on your performance including your manner and body language. Such comments are usually constructive and objective, or are intended to be so. Do not be offended. Many trainees are not aware they speak more and more quickly, becoming indistinct, when they know the topic well. Some sound bored if they have answered the same question previously. Try not to be too sensitive to feedback you receive and remember, they are trying to help you. If you have persistently played with a pen or doodled during the viva (as many do), then this needs to be pointed out to you. Likewise, if you continually fiddle with your hair or drum your fingers on the desk, fidgeting like this is very distracting and creates a bad impression. While you will not fail solely by annoying the examiners, they will rely on their overall impression of your performance if they deem you to be borderline and you will not receive the benefit of the doubt.

Be receptive to coaching and remember to maintain eye contact with the examiner. Keep your hands still and speak clearly and confidently.

If you are unsure of an answer, there are several things you can do. If you have not heard or understood the question, it is acceptable to ask the examiner to repeat it or to give clarification (although the questions are worded and read so specifically that the latter is seldom required). You can state your mind has gone blank and ask if it is possible to move on to the next question for now and return to that particular question later. When you are asked a question you perceive as difficult, there are several '*do nots*' to bear in mind. Do not roll your eyes, utter profanities, sigh and look despondent, state that you can never remember this one, or confide that you hoped this would never have been asked! This is one time where honesty is not the best policy; and you will not gain favour or sympathy from the examiners by admitting you have no experience of, have not seen, nor even heard of, what you are being asked about. The questions are all less than four years old and are directly relevant to the intermediate curriculum and the practice of anaesthesia at that level.

Ignorance is not an excuse. It is reasonable to simply state 'I don't know, sorry' if you do not know the answer. If you do hazard a guess at a question that you are unsure of, your answer will not be any less wrong by saying it quietly, hesitantly, or with a questioning look at the examiner. There is no point in answering 'Is it because . . . ?' or 'I think it's due to . . . But I'm not really sure'. Such mannerisms only serve to highlight the fact that you do not know the answer. The examiner will not give you the answer, no matter how nicely you ask! Just say your answer, stop talking, and wait for the next question to be asked. If more detail is required from you, a supplementary question will be forthcoming. If you stop talking, you will avoid veering off at a tangent or digging yourself into a hole. When they do not know the answer, candidates often offer anything they do know, however tenuously it may be related to the question asked, or they spout information they may have heard yet know nothing further about. Any additional information you offer in this way risks that the examiner will pursue it further, so take care only to mention that which you can expand upon knowledgeably.

When you find gaps in your knowledge during viva practice, remedy them at the first opportunity. Do not allow them to accumulate on a list of topics 'to be learned before the exam' because I know from experience that these topics are continually postponed and are often not learned.

Following the written exam, plan to take the SOE at the next available sitting. Although the written pass is valid for three years, do not delay needlessly as this only prolongs the agony and allows your knowledge to decay back to a level requiring more than just revision. Without exception, every candidate I know who has chosen to take an extra six months off before attempting the SOE has regretted it. Have a break while you await confirmation that you have passed the written paper before starting to prepare for the next sitting of the viva. The RCoA has now ensured that any candidate passing the written paper will be accommodated in the next available round of SOEs.

If you perform badly in any one question during the viva or feel you have not done well enough to pass, you *must* keep going, regardless. If you quit midway through a question, you will receive a score of 1—a fail. Equally important is that when the subject changes, your mindset changes, too. Draw a line underneath your performance. Put your brain back to neutral. Do not dwell on what has already happened; you cannot change it but you can change what is about to happen next. You must regroup quickly and concentrate on the subsequent question. Have you ever seen Maria Sharapova quit a tennis match when she is one set down? What does she think at the beginning of the second set? Clearly, she does not continue to bemoan losing the previous set or berate herself on her lack of performance. No, she is looking ahead with her eye on the prize, knowing that it is still her match to win or lose. It is your viva. Only you can cause yourself to fail. Do not give up before the final bell rings.

The Final SOE is in two sections: Viva 1 is the clinical viva and lasts for 50 minutes; Viva 2 is on the application of basic science to anaesthesia, intensive care, and pain management.

Viva 1a: clinical long case

The clinical long case may come from any part of the 2010 Intermediate Curriculum but bear in mind that each exam is balanced to ensure that all areas of the curriculum are sampled. Therefore, units of training which were not tested in the written paper will appear in the SOE, either as a long clinical case or as one of the short clinical cases. This may help you to direct your studying in the days preceding the exam.

You will have 10 minutes alone to read the clinical history and relevant information pertaining to the clinical case, before you meet the examiners. You can expect there will be some blood test results from biochemistry or haematology, or arterial blood gases. Often, there will be an ECG or a chest X-ray, or sometimes both. You should read the question carefully and plan your answer during this time. Commonly, the examiners will begin by asking you to 'Summarize the case' or 'Tell me about the case' and you should prepare and practise your answer to this in advance. A clear, concise, and succinct opening sentence, outlining the important facts and delivered smoothly will make an excellent first impression on the examiners and will make you feel confident and calm.

The viva element will last approximately 20 minutes and usually progresses through a discussion about the pre-operative, intra-operative, and post-operative management of the patient. There may be a critical incident at some point and there may be a complication of surgery or anaesthesia. Try to anticipate these questions during the initial 10 minutes thinking time. You should ask yourself, 'What are they likely to ask about this case?'.

You will be asked how you are going to anaesthetize the patient. You must answer the question and state how you would do this. This sounds obvious, but when faced with an incredibly difficult case in the viva, many candidates delay and delay and never get around to putting the patient off to sleep! Here you have to strike a balance between the 'driving test' mode of answering, including the routine basics and minimal standards expected (monitoring, intravenous access, and assistance), and getting to the point of actually anaesthetizing the patient. You will not pass the viva by postponing the case while you 'take a careful history and examine the respiratory system' or continue to check more and more equipment.

If the examiner has to drag the answer from you, prompt you to move on, and ask repeatedly what you would do next, you will proceed very slowly and may not get through all parts of the question and, therefore, will be unable to score maximal points. Extensive prompting in this way also merits a borderline score.

It may be the hardest thing in the world to do, but do try to relax. Try to relax and imagine the case in question. Think about how you actually do these cases or have done them in the past. If you have not seen one or done one, think back over your reading on the subject. What did you learn about it? Think about similar cases you do have experience of and apply basic principles to the case in question. Think about what you would do if faced with such a case on call one night. What plans would you make? What aspects would you discuss with your consultants? What information would you ask for from the surgeons? What difficulties would you anticipate? What else might be important? Alternatively, imagine you are in the coffee room discussing the same case. You might think aloud or ask some questions of others. You can do this in the exam too: if you do not know the answer in this part of the exam, you must show you have a sensible plan to proceed. If you are going to discuss the case with a senior, do so in a logical fashion. Explain how you would communicate the case (use the situation, background, assessment and recommendation (SBAR) system or similar) and be explicit in stating the level of help you are requesting.

If it is a case you do have experience of, try to relax and imagine how you would explain the decisions you are making to a new start in anaesthetics or to a medical student in your theatre. There may be several correct answers to a clinical problem and, in this exam, you must show that in your anaesthetic plan you have considered all the options available (even if only to discount those with which you are not familiar), before providing a reason for choosing one. This will show your breadth of knowledge and your ability to use this to manage a particular case. This is one area of the exam where clinical experience, or lack thereof, is particularly obvious.

Remember you are talking theoretically about a clinical case, you are not actually doing it! Do not hesitate, for instance, if you think the patient really needs an awake fibreoptic intubation or an upper limb block, but you are not confident in your ability to do these techniques. There is no need to mention you have only ever seen one of these and it did not work! Say you will prepare your equipment and provide topical anaesthesia to the airway or will identify the plexus using ultrasound, and so on. These techniques 'work' in vivas in a way they do not in real life. You should, however, have a plan B, should the examiner tell you your technique of choice does not work.

Viva 1b: short clinical cases

The final 20 minutes of the morning viva is allocated to three short clinical cases that will be asked by the second examiner. These may come from any area of the 2010 Intermediate Curriculum and again, remember that the exam is balanced to sample all areas in at least one component of the exam. Large topics that did not appear in the SAQ paper are very likely to be examined in the clinical viva.

These cases may involve artefacts, too, and there is a computer monitor at each station used to display X-rays, photographs, or pictures. You may ask for an investigation as part of a clinical case and be shown the result on the screen. In the clinical cases, you will plan to pass each question by showing you are a competent, confident clinician with a range of skills and experience which you can call upon to determine the most appropriate care for the patient in question. It is acceptable to ask for 'senior help' or a 'second pair of hands' if the case is of a severe enough nature to warrant this. You are not expected to know everything but you are expected to know what you require from senior help.

Viva 2

This lasts for 30 minutes and consists of four questions on applied basic science, intensive care, or pain management. Each examiner will ask two questions.

You must tread a fine line between answering the questions completely, not digging any holes for yourself, and avoiding the need for repeated prompting from the examiner. The close marking system means that for each viva you will be awarded two marks for a pass, one for borderline, and zero for a fail, by each examiner. You need 32 marks (out of a possible 40) to pass, and therefore in the whole day, you can only afford to get eight borderline marks awarded or four fails. This equates to four and two questions respectively, as each is marked independently by both examiners. If the examiners have to prompt and cajole every bit of information they want from you, it will show that you are hesitant and reticent, and it will be assumed this is because you have no belief in your knowledge. In this situation, you are more than likely to be marked borderline, even if you get to the answer eventually. It is your viva and you should be doing most of the talking.

CHAPTER 11

Summary

One day at a conference, I spent a pleasant lunchtime speaking to a man I had never met before about many of the challenges facing candidates studying for the FRCA. He told me he had left school at 16 years of age and began a steady, secure job in engineering. Sixteen years later, aged 32, he saw that engineering companies in the UK were closing and that his company was probably no exception to this. He decided he wanted to do better in life. He had a wife and children by this stage, and studied an array of job advertisements to find the ideal second career for him. He decided accountancy fitted the bill and began his studies later in life, at significant opportunity cost to him and his family. I asked him how he studied effectively with a family and other commitments. He told me his wife banished him to the shed to study for his professional accountancy exams. He was not allowed out; she would bring him flasks of coffee, while he continued to work. There were no distractions in the shed. His time was precious and he used it well, passing his exams and becoming a qualified accountant. He subsequently became an examiner for his accountancy body's final exam. This motivated man was the then Chief Executive of the RCoA.

The building blocks of success

Success in postgraduate exams requires more than knowledge alone. Figure 11.1 shows again the very simplistic fish-bone diagram first seen in Chapter 2. Instead of highlighting the issues contributing to a problem or undesirable outcome, it can be interpreted in reverse, to show those domains which must be managed optimally to culminate in exam success.

Note that knowledge forms the backbone and represents the foundations of exam success. The confounding 'bones' will each carry different emphasis for individuals, but recognize that each one always has some bearing on the overall outcome. Armed with this knowledge, you can devise a strategy of exam preparation which utilizes and takes advantage of all these confounding variables. Doing so will allow your knowledge to fall into place and will give you a deep-rooted confidence that you are well prepared.

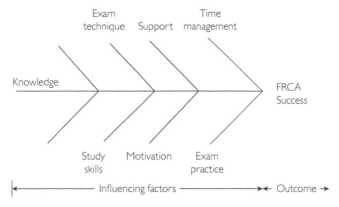

Figure 11.1 Fish-bone diagram: factors influencing exam outcome.

Plan to pass

The widely used quote paraphrased as 'To fail to plan is to plan to fail' has been attributed to many great orators and wise men in the past. It remains true in many aspects of life today and none more so than in postgraduate professional exams. The way to pass these exams is to plan to pass, prepare to pass, and practice to pass, leaving nothing to chance.

Index